Dr. Finneson on Low Back Pain

Dr. Finneson
on
Low Back Pain

Bernard E. Finneson, MD

with

Arthur S. Freese

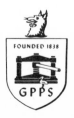

G. P. PUTNAM'S SONS, *New York*

SBN: 399-115337-4
Library of Congress Catalog Card Number: 75-15342

PRINTED IN THE UNITED STATES OF AMERICA

To our respective wives, Barbara and Ruth,
in appreciation of their forbearance and support
both here and through the years

CONTENTS

INTRODUCTION:
What This Book Has for You— and Who Dr. Finneson Is
By Arthur S. Freese

WE ARE talking about what has become the worst plague of the twentieth century, for back problems are replacing the common cold as our most frequent malady and have always been both more disabling and more agonizing than colds. It's a problem which hits the headlines often—strikes President and Senator, glamorous movie star and famous athlete, the illustrious and the humble, the stevedore and the deskbound office worker alike with a democratic and total impartiality. In all it affects more than one in every three Americans, men, women and children. In nine out of ten cases the pain and problems are located in the low back.

One sufferer is brought into the hospital on a stretcher, in such pain that should anyone place a hand too roughly on the stretcher the patient will cry out in agony. Other victims may have a pins-and-needles feeling of leg or foot or numbness or even loss of use of the limb. There are those who develop stiff frozen spines and are unable to bend or twist their backs. Some may have their chest expansion in breathing sharply curtailed, while others suffer difficulty in urinating or defecating, with constipation sometimes the first signal of a major emergency. There are those who take to bed or sofa virtually the whole day, while others have a loss of height or display a hunchbacked or swaybacked appearance. There may be a tendency to trip over little unevennesses—curbs or rocks or the edge of a carpet.

11

The most feared aspect of low back problems is the pain—often a chronic intractable menace which in its worst forms becomes terribly destructive, altering the sufferer's personality and turning an active young adult into a chronic invalid or a cripple. Even in its milder forms this never-ending pain can tear at and degrade the very quality of life. The torment can take away happiness and enjoyment, limiting the victims in all their activities from sports to driving, from lifting up a baby to standing on line for a movie or sitting in the stands at a football game.

As for the low back, you don't need any expert to explain this to you: It's simply the part of the back below the level of the ribs, a section distinctly different from any other.

Causes and Treatments of Low Back Pain

The causes are many and varied, but in general, back problems are the price people pay for their success in the long evolutionary race, for their coming down out of the trees and learing to walk upright. In addition, the individual may suffer for his failure to succeed in the everyday problems of living. The cause of any particular backache may vary from ordinary simple overuse, abuse or nervous tension to those rarer instances which demand complex delicate neurological surgery or may be life-threatening conditions involving some of the most terrible and frightening diseases known.

Treatments, too, cover a broad range, utilizing many different methods and modalities. These vary from the most ancient therapies, such as heat or cold or massage, to the latest complex products of Space Age technology. There are sophisticated electronic devices only a half dozen years old whose electrodes are implanted directly on that very delicate spinal cord itself. Here electrical impulses are beamed through the skin to be transmitted to the spinal cord electrodes, which somehow short-circuit and block the pain impulses ordinarily carried by the spinal nerve to the brain, where the hurt is "felt."

Doctors have turned to nature for the juice of a strange exotic tropical fruit for spinal injections which may soon make obsolete one of the most dangerous and demanding of spinal operations. And there's Dr. Finneson's innovation, the low back pain clinic, which will, it is hoped, open the way to a more concentrated expertise and a greater understanding with increased help for the victims of low back disorders.

Back pain and problems have led to brilliant and innovative surgery—as well as, unfortunately, to large numbers of unnecessary operations. Many patients have been surgically mutilated for no purpose; others have been turned into drug addicts as a result of the medical profession's failure in the handling of chronic pain. Here then are the many facets of these low back problems.

What This Book Is All About

This book is meant to help you: to explain what your back is like and how it got that way; what goes wrong with the low back and what can be done to treat it; how you can prevent trouble and what you can do for its difficulties. You'll also learn which doctor or specialist is best for these problems and how to judge his qualifications. If you're advised to undergo surgery, you'll learn the ways to double-check whether you should have an operation (something you should *always* confirm) and to ascertain whether the surgeon is qualified.

When a physician offers this sort of advice, you want to know something about him. The nearly half million MDs in the United States range all the way from the brilliant innovative heart surgeon Dr. Denton Cooley and the late beloved Dr. Paul Dudley White to the West Coast surgeon recently reported guilty of some forty unnecessary or bungled back operations. Some physicians become medical scientists working in isolated experimental laboratories far from any patients; others carry out administrative tasks in a wide variety of fields.

Many physicians have given up the actual practice of medicine in order to work in widely differing areas. One abandoned his medical specialty to become a practicing psychic; others have turned to writing (like Dr. Walter Alvarez, the medical columnist, or Drs. Frank Slaughter and A. J. Cronin, the novelists), while still others have become business executives, even world-famous oil magnates or astronauts.

So the possession of an MD degree doesn't really tell you very much about the owner's knowledge of medicine. But here are the facts about our author that make what he has to say of particular importance to you for your medical well-being.

Who Is Dr. Finneson?

Dr. Bernard E. Finneson has long been known to the medical profession as a successful neurosurgeon, an associate professor of neurological surgery at Philadelphia's Hahnemann Medical College, the chief of neurological surgery at three major Pennsylvania hospitals and a member of prestigious specialty medical societies. He has had five medical textbooks published here and abroad—these cover his deep and long interest in a variety of pain problems; his latest text is devoted solely to the low back.

Dr. Finneson practices medicine in the finest Hippocratic tradition. While leading the way into the medical practice of the future, he is still living and working in the traditions of the old-time family doctor, the GP of beloved memory. For Finneson is truly a "doctor" in the full sense of that word, a tradition now lost to the medical profession as a whole and rescued only by a dedicated few.

Dr. Finneson abandoned a lucrative and busy neurosurgery practice to devote his entire time to a specialty so new it doesn't even have an official name. And he's (so far as he knows) the first and only specialist in low back problems, or dysfunctions, as doctors term them. He is pioneering because "low back pain is one of the most common plagues of modern man, and if I can make a contribution—make a dent in the problem—it'll all have been worth it." He also founded the Low Back Pain Clinic (the first but no longer the only one of its kind) at Crozer-Chester Medical Center, whose hospital facilities compare favorably with those of the largest metropolitan centers.

Dr. Finneson's first concern is his patient's welfare. This neurosurgeon can be found at his hospital at 7 A.M. or so on weekdays—to operate on or to see his patients, to perform tests, which as we shall see later, can be carried out only there. He visits there, too, on Saturdays and Sundays: "Any patient who is sick has a right to be seen by his doctor—and on weekends and holidays as well." When he has office hours—on Tuesdays and Thursdays—they begin at 11 A.M., after hospital rounds, and go right through without lunch until 9 or 10 P.M.

The time he devotes to each patient is in the old tradition—as much as is needed, even if it runs to an hour or two, and he drives his secretary to distraction.

What in his background made him this way when the medical profession in general is so different?

THE YOUNG DOCTOR

Bernard Finneson was accepted by three medical schools, including Hahnemann Medical College in Philadelphia. He chose the latter because his family was poor and he could live at home. He got his MD in 1948 and says, "The first car in our family came only after I became a doctor and needed one."

Right from the start the human brain intrigued him, and he followed his Philadelphia internship with a psychiatric residency (an advanced internship, in a specialty) in New York City. In the 1940s this field was really a mixed bag— neuropsychiatry it was (and still is) called—involving both neurology (the study of nervous system disorders) and psychiatry. The young doctor was depressed by those pretranquilizer days: "The cure rate then was probably not much better than in the days of Bedlam, the first madhouse established in 1547 in London, when a certain percentage of people did get better—and this cure rate was still about the same when I was a psychiatric resident."

But in neurology he found clean, sharp guidelines—he could tell from a stroke's symptoms and his tests exactly where the problem in the brain lay. So he found himself, of necessity, working closely with neurosurgeons. When the Bronx Veterans Administration Hospital needed a neurosurgery resident, he applied and was appointed in 1950. Two years later he was called up for Army service during the Korean conflict. According to Dr. Finneson, "Doctors are a valuable commodity in the Army, and they don't like to upset you. They offered to assign me to a hospital in Philadelphia. But there's no hunger like the hunger of the neurosurgery resident for surgery. The operations you watch are long and arduous—you do nothing, just watch, until you're sure you can do it better than that guy operating there (you can't, but you're sure you can). To make matters worse, neurosurgeons are even less generous with work than other surgeons. I remember one five-hour-long operation where I was masked, gloved and gowned, and at the end I was handed a few cutoff sutures to drop in the wastebasket—my total contribution."

The young surgeon quickly volunteered for conflict—and some neurosurgery. He was shipped to Korea so fast that he never finished his indoctrination courses, never learned to salute or read a map. It took three months for his uniforms to catch up with him, and meanwhile, he had to make do with a pair of tan slacks and a golf sweater. In Korea he was in the original MASH, the Mobile Army Surgical Hospital, where in two years he gained more neurosurgical experience than he would have had in six or eight years of civilian life.

While in Korea and later in Japan, he learned about acupuncture from its Oriental practitioners at a time when it was virtually unknown in America. Coming back in early 1955, he completed his residency, took his "boards" (we'll explain this in the chapter on choosing your doctor), and as a recognized specialist began practice with an older neurosurgeon in Pennsylvania.

HOW DR. FINNESON CAME TO THE LOW BACK

To explain Dr. Finneson's interest in the lower back, we must backtrack to 1950 and his VA neurosurgery residency. After World War II the VA was plagued with hordes of veterans claiming service-connected low back dysfunctions which could cost the government vast amounts of disability payments. In desperation the VA set up a Low Back Pain Evaluation Board to diagnose causes and improve treatment.

At that time the VA allowed only neurosurgeons to operate on back problems, so it was only natural that the neurosurgery resident—then Bernard Finneson—was appointed to this new low back board. "At first this was a chore, but then I found myself caught up in the problems, and so, as far back as 1950, I was devoting a disproportionately large amount of my time to low back dysfunction and pain, and this carried over into my private practice."

The older neurosurgeon with whom Dr. Finneson became associated had one of the very large Pennsylvania practices and naturally gave Finneson all cases dealing with back problems. Out of this concentrated and large experience came Dr. Finneson's first and highly regarded medical textbook, *Diagnosis and Management of Pain Syndromes* (a syndrome is a group of characteristic symptoms of a particular disorder), in 1962. A Spanish-language edition followed, and then an entirely new and revised edition of both versions in 1969. Finally, in 1973 came his latest textbook, *Low Back Pain,* which was enthusiastically greeted by the medical profession.

Clinics and private practitioners specializing in pain problems find that three-quarters and more of the sufferers they see center their complaints on the low back. Yet until Finneson's clinic there was no concentrated work being done on the low back, and this disturbed the neurosurgeon. He gradually phased out his general neurosurgical practice, leaving only the low back sufferers. "I didn't want to dilute my knowledge by having to think about headaches or facial pain or the latest surgical techniques for tic douloureux or the like because no one can be the best of all things—the best tumor surgeon, the best neurosurgeon, the best spinal disk surgeon and so on. To be the best in one field is a matter of experience, of commitment, of zeroing in in your own mind so that the area is all you think about each day. And finally I felt that to be expert enough to warrant the referrals I was getting from other neurosurgeons and doctors, I should limit myself to this one field."

Dr. Finneson became the first specialist in the low back. At his Low Back Pain Clinic he sees everyone, and free clinic patients sit side by side with the wealthy: "I didn't want a clinic with hard wooden benches and free patients waiting in droves while I quickly finished and went to my exquisitely appointed private office with its rich patients. My clinic *is* my office—whoever calls first gets the first appointment; we never ask whether he's a private patient or a free one."

More than anything else, Dr. Finneson is open-minded. "If I hear of anyone who has something to say which might be relevant to what I'm doing, I want to listen, and I'll go wherever that doctor is. If I think the new idea or technique is applicable to my own low back work, I'll try to learn it. If it's not usable, I'll just forget the whole thing."

It's in this spirit that he has written this book—to provide the latest knowledge and the most practical help possible, along with an understanding of the problem, so that *you* can use the information to get the best available help.

I'm proud to have had the opportunity to help in this task, and I shall now let Dr. Finneson speak for himself, for it is his wisdom and knowledge that can help you. The "I" from here on refers to Dr. Finneson himself.

Part I

The Basic Facts on Your Low Back

Chapter 1

THE CAUSE OF YOUR TROUBLES:
How Your Back Got That Way

In a very real sense our aching backs are a two-legged problem! For rodents, too, develop aching backs and slipped disks like ours when we make them walk about on two legs. One Neanderthal man who lived almost 100,000 years ago near Düsseldorf, Germany, also suffered backaches. We will go into the details of these cases—significant in tracking down the cause of our low back problems—at the end of this chapter. First, let's look at man himself and how his aching back came about, for he didn't have one before he actually became man. For this understanding we have to turn the clock back to when the world was truly young, to see how human development came about—an evolutionary rat race (in the very sense in which we use the phrase today), a struggle to outdistance fellow creatures, to shove others aside in order to seize the good things of life. Out of it all, nature struggled to develop a better animal, which is what man would like to be.

When our ancestors were still half ape, half human, they developed from four-legged into two-legged primates—but they paid a price (which we still pay) in the form of low back problems. Man's larger brain and his ability to use his hands for everything from throwing a spear to producing an exquisite painting or writing a love sonnet were all developed, but in the process defects appeared as humans did things nature had neither anticipated nor provided for. The upright stature brought with it the aching backs, the abdominal hernias

21

and the varicose veins, the hemorrhoids and the flat feet. Each time any of us is bothered by one of these problems he is actually bearing silent witness to the stresses of the erect position, proof that nature hadn't fully planned for this new creature who somehow moved ahead almost on his own, discarding the processes by which nature developed other animals.

We'll be talking more of primates, so let's clarify the term. It comes from the Latin *primas,* which means one of the first, and reflects man's own view of himself. For the term "primate" is applied to what is considered the highest order of mammals, including the apes, monkeys, lemurs—and man himself, of course.

My interest in this postural evolution was originally excited by a Fundamentalist minister whom I treated for low back problems. I made the mistake of commenting that all these problems really began when our ancestors first came crawling out of the primeval slime, out of the oceans where life first began. When these early animals moved onto dry land, they started the long evolutionary process that was to lead through four-legged animals to those that lived in trees. When these tree dwellers eventually came down to run about the earth on two legs instead of four, they initiated the changes that led to slipped disks and aching backs.

However, this explanation precipitated an impassioned and lively lecture from the minister to convince me that evolution was only an ill-conceived, unproved and thoroughly mistaken theory. Challenged, I had no choice but to seek out the proof he questioned, to be sure I *was* right. As a matter of fact, the whole reconstruction of evolution, with its probing of man's own roots represents one of our greatest scientific achievements, and only a few months ago, in the heart of Ethiopia, a joint American-French-Ethiopian team of anthropologists (headed by a professor from Cleveland's Case Western Reserve University) found upper and lower fossil jaws which likely date man's own beginnings back to almost 5,000,000 years ago.

If anything warrants the name of "scientific magic," it's the way anthropologists take fossil fragments and from these bits of tooth or bone proceed to reconstruct not only the skeleton of the ancient creature, but even its life-style and the kind of existence it led when the earth was still young. Typical of this strange detective work was the unearthing in 1927 of a single fossil molar from a cave in the limestone hills at Choukoutien, thirty miles from Peking, China.

For hundreds of years the Chinese had known of the presence of these ancient bones and had been crudely digging them out to grind up and sell for the powder's supposed medicinal and magical effects. It's heartbreaking to think how many rare anthropological finds and treasures must have disappeared forever down the gullets of countless dyspeptic Chinese mandarins, their wives and mistresses and courtiers.

In 1927 Dr. Davidson Black, a Canadian anthropologist, was teaching anatomy at Peking Medical College. When he was shown something unearthed from these caves, he recognized it to be a fossil molar. On the basis of this single ancient tooth he announced confidently that he had uncovered a hitherto-unknown variety of early man. With his fossil molar carefully secured in a gold locket attached to his watch chain—and with his expenses underwritten by Rockefeller Foundation funds—he moved in on that limestone pit, which was deep enough to swallow a fifteen-story apartment building.

For two years, under Dr. Black's close supervision, tons of earth were moved and sifted, but the fossil fragments turned up proved of little value and added nothing to scientific knowledge. Then a skull was found buried in a limestone bed. It took the anthropologist four months of work with the finest picks and most delicate brushes to tease that skull out from its stone bed. Only then began a meticulous, painstaking study to identify what finally proved to be a classic find. This fossil became known as the Peking Man and by itself made the entire project scientifically worthwhile.

Actually it only takes the shape of a fossil molar, the curve of a jaw, the formation of a piece of a thighbone for anthropologists to know whether the creature was a meat eater or a vegetarian, ape or ape-man or early man, whether it walked on two legs or on four, what its life-style was like. These early primates lived in the trees, for protection from the powerful wild animals that roamed the earth. Their diet was basically vegetarian.

The early primates remained in their trees for long periods, sleeping and resting there to be secure from the animals that preyed on them. To do this, the tree primates had to learn to sit and even to sleep with their bodies in an upright position rather than sprawled out on all fours—and this was the starting point for our two-legged posture. To climb a tree, primates extend their hind limbs into a position which is very close to the one you and I take in walking today.

Somewhere along his evolutionary path, man's precursor began to use his hands and arms for tools. To free his hands for this use, it became necessary for preman to walk upright. In addition, by walking on two legs, he could see over the tops of bushes and wild grasses to spot dangerous animals before they could get close enough to attack.

Moreover, two-legged walking is ideal for covering the many miles essential for hunting and is much better suited to both this and his other tasks than, for example, the chimpanzee's ability to run much faster or the monkey's capacity for outsprinting man. While gorillas, chimps and monkeys will occasionally stand with bent knees for short periods, this is neither a habitual nor a customary posture. Only man stands straight upright, and the resultant forward curvature of his low back spine differentiates him from all other primates and is simultaneously the cause of his backaches.

A combination of evolutionary success and evolutionary failure have produced man's backaches. At some point, the continuous primeval forests began to break up; the trees separated into groves and clumps rather than one unending stretch covering the entire dry land. This change forced the tree-dwelling animals to fight for the now-limited leafy space. The losers took to the ground to seek another clump of trees, whose inhabitants they now had to fight in an effort to claim living room in this new haven.

Eventually the diminishing trees of the forests became populated by the more powerful, the more successful animals. The weaker ones, the evolutionary failures, got along either on the ground around the trees or in the flatlands between the disappearing forests. The trees were won by the ancestors of the gorilla and chimpanzee, while early man or preman was actually an evolutionary failure. Driven out of his home, he was forced to find some means of survival on the ground. The result was a two-legged existence for which nature had not designed this animal, this man, and for which he was to pay dearly.

Unlike the spines of his animal relatives, man's spine is no longer straight (as we shall discuss in the next chapter). The human spine curves, dipping forward in the abdominal or low back area, curving backward in the chest section and then forward once more as it stretches upward into the neck, where it supports the weight of the head. With these changes, the whole center of gravity shifted frontward, and an exclusively human development appeared—our buttock muscles balance out this forward shift in the body. Coming late in evolution, these changes have produced our back problems.

Since animals don't stand upright ordinarily, they aren't bothered with back trouble. However, the bulldog, the beagle and the dachshund are plagued by back problems—but only because they are actually achondroplastic dwarfs. Like some humans, these particular dogs have a growth defect in the cartilage of their long bones and their development is stunted. This inherited problem also leads to a narrowing of the dog's spinal canals, causing back dysfunctions which would be felt as pain in man.

In fact, there really isn't that much difference between the spines of dogs and humans. The essential difference isn't in the spine, but in the way it functions or works. In four-legged animals the spine acts as a suspension bridge with fore and hind limbs acting as piers supporting the structure at its two ends. In these animals the body is virtually hanging down from the spine, which is slung fairly straight from hind to fore limbs. As we will see in the next chapter, the flowing curvatures of the human spine develop and change as the fetus grows into the child and then on into adolescence and eventual adulthood.

The final and ultimate proof that the upright position is the real culprit in our backaches has come from an intriguing experiment with rodents at Tokushimo University Medical School in Japan. Here Dr. Kengo Yamada produced a sort of "instant postural evolution." He amputated the forelegs and tails of rats and mice on the third to the seventh day after birth—and produced sixty-two rats and fifty-three mice (a quarter of the total newborn) that gradually developed the ability to stand and walk about in a semi-erect posture.

Walk like a human being, and evidently you can expect to suffer backaches like a human being as well. For X rays of the spines of these two-legged rodents showed that instead of their normal straight spines, they developed an abnormal forward curvature of the low back spine such as human beings often suffer.

In addition, microscopic spinal studies revealed that the changes occurring in the rodent's spinal disks resembled those normally occurring with age in the human being. The rats and mice even suffered actual slipped or herniated disks. Even the osteoarthritis which most humans develop after the age of forty appeared among these animals. Incidentally, not a single slipped or herniated disk was found in those animals which had not undergone amputation but had continued their usual four-legged existences.

We can only assume that these two-legged mice and rats with their slipped disks and their arthritis—like their human counterparts—must have felt equivalent pain and suffered with similar aching backs. In any case, here is actual experimental proof of the fact that back problems and slipped disks are the price of the upright position, the two-legged posture. Nearly 100,000 years ago Neanderthal man suffered with these disabilities. In fact, it's because of his back problems that we have the warped and distorted picture that is conventionally held of this early man. In 1856 some quarry workers stumbled on a skullcap and some limbs from a cave in the limestone cliffs of the Neander Valley (*Neanderthal* in German) near Düsseldorf, Germany.

This proved to be the first human fossil to be recognized as such, and a number of the experts of that time identified the remains as early man. Beetle-browed with large cheeks and a receding chin, Neanderthal man (as the fossil and his fellows were then named) had a brain about as large as ours. He was about five feet tall, had a powerful frame, short stubby hands and feet, and was heavy-muscled and very strong.

On the basis of this first-found fossil, Neanderthal man is still usually pictured as not quite erect, almost hunchbacked, in fact. He's commonly shown as standing or shuffling about his world with bent knees—a squat, stooping, brutish and somewhat apelike creature. Only none of this happens to be true. It's all a misconception produced and perpetuated because of the bad back of one sufferer of this early breed of man. For the only Neanderthal man skeleton with an almost complete spine was the one that's been popularly known as "the old man of La Chapelle-aux-Saints."

Only in recent years has the reexamination and careful study of this famous skeleton revealed that the poor devil's spine was actually markedly deformed. He had suffered the ravages of an extensive and severe arthritic condition which even today is the most common form of this disorder— hypertrophic osteoarthritis, the arthritis of wear and tear, the results of use. Perhaps this particular individual lived a lot longer than we are likely to think about where early man is concerned and so felt the effects of a long and what must have been a hard life.

In actuality, the Neanderthal man was completely erect and not at all apelike. In fact, if a healthy one of his fellows were shaved and his hair cut in any approved fashion, dressed in a pair of slacks and a sports shirt, he would probably not even be unduly conspicuous today if he joined a crowd at the ball game or went shopping on a Saturday afternoon—although he might seem a bit short and certainly very powerful. But he would clearly be as likely as the rest of us to suffer with an aching back.

Chapter 2

THE LOWDOWN ON YOUR BACK:
What's There and How It Works

DESPITE ALL the trouble your back may be giving you or
the amount it gives all people, your back is really constructed
about as well as any other major part or organ of your body.
But like your heart, which is cheated of exercise, or given a
high-fat diet, like your stomach subjected to frequent emotional upsets or constant anger, your back will cause you
problems. Before we go into the problems and what you can
do for them, we must first understand what's beneath it all—
the bones, muscles, ligaments and nerves of your back, how
they develop and the ways they must work together for your
back to do its job.

Your Backbone: How It Began

A week after the egg has been fertilized in the mother's
uterus the embryo comes into contact with the uterine wall
and sticks to it. Digesting the lining tissue at this point, the
embryo embeds itself, and the miracle of growth is under
way. The sixteen-day-old embryo already contains the back's
precursor—a clump of cells soon to form the notochord,
which will later persist as the gellike center of the spinal
disks.

By three weeks the somites or primitive segments, are
clearly defined on both sides of the growing spine. The somites look like so many kernels on an ear of corn, and the
spinal nerves now appear in this area, along with the precur-

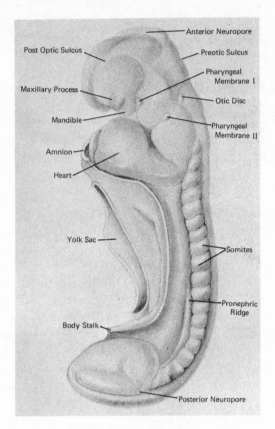

Figure 1. At three or four weeks the surface landmarks become recognizable.

sors of the vertebrae (the bones forming the spine). Steadily the vertebrae grow and take final shape, while the intervertebral or spinal disks also take shape and form. Actually these will continue to change—particularly the disks—steadily and gradually throughout life.

In the fetus or very young child there are actually thirty-three separate vertebrae, but by adulthood those at the very base of the spine will have fused (forming the sacrum and coccyx, of which we will talk shortly), and there will then be only twenty-six separate vertebrae.

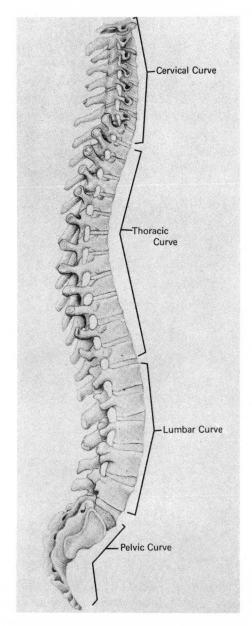

Figure 2. Lateral view of the vertebral column.

The Spinal Column and Its Curves

In the human body the spine is divided into sections. First there is the cervical (the neck) spine, consisting of seven vertebrae; the seventh (doctors write this C7) is what you touch if you put your hand at the back of base of your neck and feel the bony prominence there. There are twelve thoracic (chest) vertebrae and five lumbar (low back) vertebrae. The lumbar begins where the ribs stop, and if you feel the tops of your hipbones and then the vertebra on a line between these crests, you will be feeling L4, the fourth and next to last lumbar vertebra. The five sacral and four coccygeal vertebrae continue down from the last lumbar vertebra. In the adult these nine bones are fused into two, the sacrum and the coc-

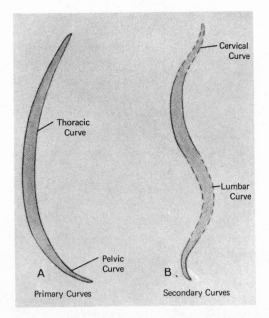

Figure 3. A, The early fetal spine, which is completely concave, embodies both the thoracic and pelvic curves; B, the secondary cervical and lumbar curves are superimposed.

cyx, and these two may even fuse with each other in later adulthood.

The human spine is distinctly curved as you view it from the side, unlike the fairly straight one of quadrupeds. As early as three months, the fetal spine is completely concave. It actually has two curves (called primary because they are present in fetal life). One of these is the thoracic curve (from T2 to T12, or from the second to the twelfth thoracic vertebra), which is concave toward the front, while the pelvic curve begins at the junction between the last lumbar and the first sacral vertebrae and runs to the end of the coccyx, the end of the spine. The pelvic curve too is similarly concave but inclined somewhat downward.

These primary curves are provided by nature to allow room for the chest and abdominal organs in the fetus. When the infant begins to sit up at about three months of age, it develops a cervical curve (least marked of these bends and from C1 to T2). This is convex toward the front and becomes well established only at the age of four months, when the infant is capable of holding its head up. Next, the lumbar curve (from T12 to the junction of lumbar and sacral vertebrae), which is also convex anteriorly, starts to form in the first year, when the infant begins to walk. This latter curve isn't fully consolidated until adulthood.

These secondary curves are also called compensatory, for they permit the upright two-legged posture, and it has been estimated that the spinal curves make the backbone some sixteen times stronger than if it were straight. They permit the spine to transmit the weight of the body to the pelvis and reduce the muscular effort otherwise needed to keep you upright. It's the development of these curves that causes the baby's back to straighten and its bottom becomes less noticeable as it learns to walk. However, a woman's lower back is more hollowed out than a man's, and her bottom more prominent, owing to natural differences in the lumbar curve. And when she's pregnant, the lumbar curve flattens out—to be restored after delivery.

But it is the vertebrae and disks which make up the spine and its curves.

THE SPINAL BONES AND DISKS

The spinal column is nature's construction game. It's a matter of piling building blocks one atop the other, with shock absorbers between and the vertebrae held together just as guy wires hold a tower or an extension arm in position. For the spine is not a solid bone, but one made of many separate units which depend on muscles and ligaments, plus the design of the body, to keep these units from flying apart every time pressure is applied in the course of normal activity. But before we look at the biomechanics of the muscles, ligaments and nerves involved, let us examine the building blocks.

The bones of the spine vary because each section has a different job to do. Except for the sacral and coccygeal, the vertebra in general consists of a more or less massive, heavy, often kidney-shaped or roughly oval bone called the vertebral

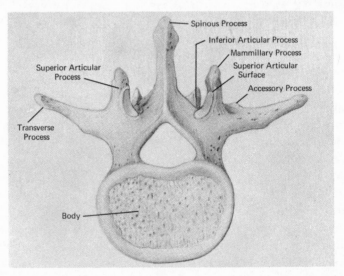

Figure 4. Cephalad view of fourth lumbar vertebra.

body. From this and extending backward, is a Y-shaped bone which encloses the delicate spinal cord, whose protection is one of the chief purposes of the spinal or vertebral column. The tail of the Y is the spinous process, and you can feel it if you run your hand down the spine—these processes are the series of sharp bones you feel along the backbone.

From each of the angled arms of the Y, and at right angles, juts another sharp spur of bone, the transverse process. Finally, pointing upward and downward on each side of the Y—between spinous and transverse processes—are four short fingers of bone terminating in smooth oval faces which form joints with (articulate with) and fit against similar faces on the next vertebrae, two against the upper and two against the lower. These are the articular facets, joints which sit like so many roof shingles on every one of the twenty-six adult vertebrae from the head to the tail of the vertebral column.

The vertebrae vary with the section. The seven cervical, or neck, vertebrae are smaller than the others, and their chief job is to provide for the movement and support of the head. In fact, the first one—C1—is called the atlas, for it carries the weight of the head on its shoulders (like the Titan Atlas of Greek mythology, who was condemned to support the heavens on his shoulders). Actually the atlas has no body, but a shelf which pivots about a peglike extension of C2, which appropriately is called the axis. From here down, the other cervical vertebrae are fairly typical except that they are on the small side and designed for mobility rather than weight bearing.

Below the cervical come the thoracic vertebrae, the first nine of which have additional smooth facets on both body and transverse processes. These extra facets articulate with the ribs, which sweep around to form joints with the sternum, or breastbone, in front. As a result, the ribs act as bracing struts for the thoracic vertebrae; this solid support is in contrast with the cervical and lumbar vertebrae, which are supported by soft tissues and so are more susceptible to damage from injuries and stress.

However, the T10 body articulates with only one rib, and T11 and T12 have facets on the body, but not their transverse processes. The ribs attached to T11 and T12 are the so-called floating ribs, for they don't attach to the breastbone in front. Larger than the cervical vertebrae, these thoracic ones are smaller than the lumbar. With their rib connections they are also relatively immobile, but they do help provide a rigid protective cage to enclose and protect the lungs and heart.

And now we come to the low back with all its problems—and its five massive lumbar vertebrae. These are the power-houses of the spine—and its Achilles' heel as well. Very heavy vertebral bodies are needed here because you concentrate an enormous workload on this very short area. In fact, when you straighten up from a bent-over position, you're using the lumbosacral spine as a fulcrum and throwing a potential force of more than a quarter of a ton into this region. Lift an object from this same position, and you're multiplying the weight by a leverage factor of from 12 to 16, depending on your height and the position of your arms.

The body of the lumbar vertebra is kidney-shaped, wider from side to side than from front to back. The space in the Y (the continuous spinal canal) where the spinal cord is lodged is small and decreases as it moves down the spine until the nerves become particularly susceptible to any pressure from a slipped disk because there is no extra room for the nerve to move aside in the L5 and S1 nerve roots.

The last of the lumbar vertebrae articulates with the sacrum in the adult where the five sacral vertebrae are fused into a single large triangular bone that is proportionately broader in man than in the animal, probably nature's compensation for the upright position. It is wedged into the pelvis, where it forms a keystone between spine and legs. The sacrum is wider in women than in men, and since with the hipbones it forms the pelvic girdle, it produces a wider pelvis for pregnancy and delivery. A channel runs through the sacrum to contain the sacral nerves.

The coccyx remains of four original vertebrae and is commonly a solid bone which in the adult is often fused to the sacrum. The coccyx is probably all that's left of what was once your tail when man was preman or even earlier in his development.

From the C2 down to the lumbosacral joint the bones do not actually touch except for the fingerlike contacts of the articular facets. For the bodies of the vertebrae are separated by that strange but effective little device, the intervertebral or spinal disk.

THE SPINAL DISKS

The disks conjure up pictures of pain and surgery in most patients' minds, but they really are essential structures which ordinarily provide a trouble-free lifetime of protection and shock absorbency for the average person. They give the spine mobility, make it possible for you to bend forward and stretch backward, to twist and rotate your body, to walk without getting your head shaken up each time your heel hits the ground, to run or jump without the trauma of hitting the ground like a ton of bricks each time you come down.

The disks vary in size, with the lumbar disks the largest. Since the low back—the lumbar region—carries the heaviest burden, it's only logical to find its disks the thickest and the heaviest and its vertebrae the most massive. However, the thoracic disks are the thinnest, and this too could be anticipated since the ribs brace these vertebrae and keep them fairly rigid, limiting their degree of mobility. The cervical disks are intermediate in thickness between lumbar and thoracic, for the cervical vertebra must provide a great deal of mobility to move the head around, tilt it, etc., while carrying only limited weight.

The disks aren't the only joints between the vertebrae, for, as mentioned earlier, facet joints are present as well. Were the disks the only joints, the vertebrae would have an almost unlimited degree of mobility to the point where this might well endanger the stability of the entire spine. But the facet joints limit the independent movement of the vertebrae, and again this is done in a way that is clearly attuned to the need of the body, that fits the need of the particular section. Thus, only the cervical vertebrae below the atlas (C1) have full freedom of movement. The thoracic vertebrae with their attached ribs can move in only two directions, while the lumbar vertebrae, which must carry the heaviest load in the human being's varied activities, are controlled but allowed to move in three directions.

The disk itself, however, is built to function like a hydraulic system. The center is filled with a viscous mass—the nucleus pulposus—which is contained by a series of concentric layers of connective tissue—the annulus fibrosus—so that in cross section the disk looks like a tree stem with its annular rings and its central pulp.

The soft consistency of the nucleus pulposus permits it to transmit the forces that arise in lifting or jumping or other activities. This gel spreads the pressure uniformly over the entire surface of the vertebral bodies (for the disk fits between these adjoining bodies down the line) and so behaves like a shock absorber. Both sections—nuclear and annulus— are sandwiched and held in place between a pair of flat circular cartilaginous plates. We will have more to say about all this in the chapter on disks and their disorders.

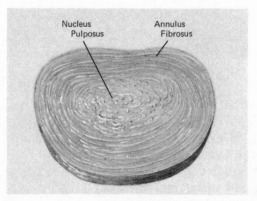

Nucleus
Pulposus

Annulus
Fibrosus

Figure 5. Sectioned lumbar intervertebral disk.

THE MOVEMENTS OF THE SPINE

We've seen how the spine is built for action, but how does it move? Basically the spine has three movements. First there is the most common, the bending forward, or flexion; allied to this is the bending sideward, or lateral flexion. The second and opposite movement is bending backward, and this is extension. Third is a simple rotation in which the spine moves about an axis drawn straight down through the bodies of the vertebrae. In short, the degree of the mobility of the spine and the way in which it moves varies with the section involved. Such movement is greatest in the cervical region and where the thoracic and lumbar or sacral and lumbar vertebrae meet (the thoracolumbar and lumbosacral junctions). The thoracic movements are the most limited because these vertebrae are tied to the ribs. Of course, all this mobility depends to a considerable extent on the muscles and ligaments of both the spine and the back.

Low Back Muscles, Ligaments and Tendons

Strange as it may seem at first glance, some of the most important low back muslces are actually in front—the abdominal muscles. Even hip and leg muscles get into the act. And of course, the low back muscles themselves are involved. Actually the greatest protection the back can have is the presence of healthy, strong, elastic muscles, ligaments and tendons.

The muscles of the back are so complex that it is difficult to determine the exact function of each one of them. There is, for example, a long strong muscle—the sacrospinalis—which runs all the way from the sacrum clear up to the skull and acts as a very powerful extensor of the spine. Like all the muscles involved, it is bilateral (on both sides of the body), and when only one of these acts, it will rotate or tilt the spine. There are other extensor muslces, some of which attach to the hip or just run from one spot on the vertebrae to another, up and down the line.

The abdominal muscles which act as flexors of the spine make it possible for you to bend your back forward or to lift your stiffened legs when you're lying on your back (a fact we use to strengthen these muscles). Working in a similar manner are muscles which run from the thighbone to the lumbar vertebrae (the psoas major and minor). These too are bilateral muscles, and if they act separately, they produce a bending sideways instead of directly forward.

These muscles are attached to the bones by tendons, very strong white glistening sheets of fibrous tissue which under ideal conditions are supple and elastic so that they can take the stresses of use. Tendons attach muscles to bones and differ from ligaments in that they hold the bones together by encapsulating joints, for example. Thus, the annulus fibrosus of the disks are formed of a dozen concentric layers, the outermost of which attaches to the vertebral bodies above and below, as well as to the broad powerful ligament (the anterior longitudinal ligament) which runs along the front of the spine from the axis to the sacrum. This ligament also attaches to the upper and lower edges of the vertebral disks so that it provides a flexible powerful link.

Another ligament runs along the back of the vertebral bodies, while others tie the transverse processes together, and still others the spinous processes. The joints too are held together by their ligaments. The ligaments hold together the many building blocks of your spine, as well as attach the sacrum and coccyx to the pelvic girdle and even the lumbar vertebrae to the pelvis.

The Nerves, Pain and the Low Back

The anatomy of pain in the low back is as complex as pain anywhere else in the body, and the problems are more involved. Here we have to deal with numbness, pins and needles and even paralysis to a greater or lesser degree. All this lies not only in the nerves in the low back but in the whole central nervous system (spinal cord and brain). So let's start at the top and work down to the local or peripheral nerves which serve the actual aching part.

The basis of the whole affair is the individual nerve cell, the neuron. Neurons can vary from microscopic in size to those which are several feet in length but less than one-hundredth of an inch in diameter (some run all the way from the feet up to the brain). In the brain, where you actually "feel" pain, there are an estimated 10 billion neurons with another 100 billion so-called glia cells.* Just one cubic inch of tissue here contains 10,000,000 cells, while a column the thickness of a pencil may contain about 50,000 neurons. No one really knows at exactly what spot in all this tangle of cells and neurons it is that we begin to "feel" pain, yet it does occur somewhere here.

Running through that continuous spinal canal in the vertebrae, the place where the Y part of the spinal column meets the vertebral bodies, is the spinal cord. A tapering cylinder of soft tissue, the spinal cord is only about a foot and a half long and has the thickness of a cigar. Nevertheless, the spine contains some 2 billion neurons and carries a never-ending two-way traffic of nerve impulses.

Sensations, including pain, run up from the body through tracts or bundles of neurons in the spinal cord to the brain, where these are interpreted and considered before necessary action is taken. The cells conducting impulses to the central nervous system are called sensory neurons. But down from the brain come others—the motor neurons—which bring orders: pull the hand away from a hot stove, lift the right leg, speed up the heart and the like. Both the sensory and the motor impulses are carried in the spinal cord.

From the spinal cord also come the so-called nerve roots which are nerves or collections of neurons splitting off from the spinal cord to supply sensations and control over the var-

*The word "glia" is derived from the Greek word meaning glue, and the function of these cells is to "glue together" or maintain in proper position the functionally active neural elements.

ious sections of the body. There are thirty-one paired spinal nerves, for these nerves come out from both sides of the spinal cord and the vertebral column to supply the two halves of the body, and each one of these nerves contains both a sensory and a motor component.

Actually the spinal column outgrows the cord. Although the cord occupies the full length of the column in early life, by adulthood the cord only reaches to the first lumbar vertebra. After this there are only those nerves that split off from the cord and through the lumbar and sacral spinal canal to reach the openings (intervertebral foramina) in the spinal column through which they will exit to reach the part of the body they supply. This collection of nerves running through the low back spinal columns is called the cauda equina, or horse's tail (which it vaguely resembles).

In order to protect this center of bodily sensation as well as body control, nature encased the spinal cord in a solid bony channel, and only after the nerves emerge through a bony opening are they exposed. This very protection is itself a danger because anything that presses against the nerves will squeeze them against unyielding bone and produce severe neurological symptoms. If you recall childhood and someone pressing your funny bone in your elbow, you'll remember the pain it caused. Actually here you're simply squeezing a main nerve against a bone—which can and does happen in the spine.

Should some of the gellike nucleus squeeze loose from the vertebral disk and press a nerve against the bony opening through which it exits—or enters—there will be a reaction. This may be the wild pain of a slipped disk irritating pain fibers, or it may be pins and needles or numbness under other circumstances (the reaction depends on which nerves in the root are affected, whether sensory or motor nerve components are most irritated or injured). Tumors will have the same effect, for the growing mass presses on the nerves adjacent to the growth, or a hemorrhage in which the volume of blood or the blood clot causes similar pressure.

Knowing the area supplied by each nerve, the doctor can tell which nerve is being compressed and so have a pretty accurate picture of the problem just, in many cases, from the patient's description alone. This will be explored in detail later in the appropriate chapters on the actual problems (such as disk and the like).

There are other roles that the so-called peripheral nerves play (peripheral nerves are those outside the central nervous system). Body tissues in general are supplied with two sets of such nerves: the sensory (to pick up sensations whether hot or cold or pain or whatever) and the motor (which carry instructions, for example, to make muscles work). When your muscles contract too much or for too long (you carry too heavy a bundle or run too far), they will begin to ache for reasons still not really understood.

If tissues—back muscles or ligaments or tendons—are injured these too will hurt. Injuring a motor nerve will produce paralysis of the part involved (a leg or the urinary bladder or any other part or organ). There may be a loss of sensation, a numbness of the part supplied, if a sensory nerve is injured.

Thus, the nerves play a major role in low back problems— but it is a complex role and one that cannot be spelled out in a few words or lines. This role is best left for the chapter devoted to the particular problem. For example, pain is not always physical, not always the "cry of an injured nerve." It may be cry of the pain of a depressed person who feels as much pain from his or her depression as from any physical injury. This too we will explore in the chapter on the psychology of low back pain.

Chapter 3

THE NEW EPIDEMIC:
An Old Disorder Turns on People

THE LOW back problems can hardly be called anything but an old disorder, for they've been around for nearly a quarter of a billion years. Nearly half a century ago, in Wyoming, Professor Roy L. Moodie unearthed a dinosaur whose tail (caudal) vertebrae had bony tumors. These growths made the animal's tail so rigid it lost its ability to move and thus perished. The first known low back problem actually proved fatal.

Considerably more recently, in the Pliocene epoch, which began some 7,000,000 years ago and lasted for about 500,000 years, preman and perhaps very early man came into being. During this period spondylitis deformans (poker back, a spinal arthritis which produces rigidity and hump-back) was widespread. And Neanderthal man, some 100,000 years ago, showed signs of spinal tuberculosis.

Although we can't be sure exactly what man was doing for his backaches then, we do know that 20,000 years ago or more Stone Age man was already drilling holes in the skulls of his fellows (trephining). This was done to relieve head-aches (often caused by tension of the neck and upper back muscles) or the pressure of fractured skulls, for epilepsy, in-sanity or even religious reasons. Surprisingly, many of these patients (or victims) survived, for we can see by their skulls that sometimes as many as five holes were drilled in a single skull with crude stone drills or knives and actually healed. This is amazing when you stop to consider that even today

44

with our sterile and gentle operating room techniques this is a dangerous operation. The Stone Age type of trephining is still being performed in virtually the same ancient way by some primitive peoples in parts of Algeria and Melanesia. The frequency of deformities and tuberculous infections of the spine before recorded history is clear from their widespread depiction in the figures used to decorate early Peruvian and North American Indian pottery. Acupuncture, too, has long been used for backaches—and since it is known to have been performed with flint or stone needles, we can only assume it, too, was practiced in the Stone Age.

The oldest of the scientific surgical texts is the Edwin Smith Surgical Papyrus, a scroll whose origins go back to the Egypt of some 5,000 years ago and whose instructions might well have been old even then. This scroll was found in a grave near Luxor, Egypt, in 1862, and Edwin Smith, an Egyptologist, purchased it in Thebes in the same year. Recognizing it as a medical text, he set it aside, and after his death, his daughter gave it to the New-York Historical Society in 1906. It was translated by James H. Breasted, who eventually published it in 1930.

This papyrus describes leg-moving tests by which the physicians of 3000 B.C. could diagnose sciatica, which even then was recognized as connected with vertebral problems. And the arthritis of the Pliocene epoch (spondylitis deformans) was common among the Egyptians (as we know from their tombs), along with osteoarthritis, especially of the sacroiliac joint. True, we're not likely today to use pig bile or the fat of a hippopotamus to treat these disorders, but we still use splints very similar to those described in this ancient papyrus.

Tuberculosis of the spine, a condition known medically as Pott's disease or tuberculous spondylitis (spondylitis is an inflammation of one or more vertebrae), was very common among the ancient Egyptians. In fact, we still see this condition, and with the reported rise of tuberculosis in our large cities it's possible we may be seeing even more of it. So widespread were these arthritic and spinal conditions among the early Egyptians that the disorders can be diagnosed by their characteristic appearance in many of their ancient statues and in their mummies. One, of a priest, Nesperehan, of 3,000 years ago, shows Pott's disease with its typical humpback.

The ancient Peruvians, too, suffered from a disease which is becoming increasingly important as we live longer, one which seems to strike the spine in particular—osteoporosis. As we shall see, we are still trying to cope with this disorder. Man has obviously suffered with his low back since he first became man and has worked to relieve his discomfort and pain with everything from braces and corsets to drugs (ancient potions utilized the aspirin family back in the Stone Age), with a generous dose of magic and suggestion added for good measure—and we're still using all these measures just as our ancestors did.

Epidemic of Pain: The Figures on Low Back Problems

There are two ways to approach these figures. First, there are the general estimates and statements, the overall impressions commonly offered; secondly, there are the detailed statistics, which in their way are even more startling than the widely used overall estimates. In addition, there are some new and still unpublished data which I've obtained from the National Center for Health Statistics of the U.S. Public Health Service.

One way of looking at this problem is to record a few of the commonly mentioned victims of backaches: President John F. Kennedy, Senator Barry Goldwater, Elizabeth Taylor and golfer Jack Nicklaus. But the most important victim is *you* or a member of your family, if one of you is among these unfortunates. Certainly you wouldn't be an exception; oft-quoted estimates are that 70,000,000 Americans have suffered with a severe backache more than once; that at least 7,000,000 receive treatment of some type for this misery every single day in the year; that 2,000,000 are added to these painful ranks every year; that 1 of very 3 adults is plagued by this pain every single day. Just to add a few dollar signs to the figures—it's estimated that at least some 200,000,000 days of work are lost from this torment every year, that it costs the United States anywhere from $1 to $10 billion annually. I've even seen it claimed that some medical textbooks contain as many as 100 or more reasons for the backaches that cause these problems.

But these are generalized summaries and estimates. Let us look at some specialized, detailed statistics of the National Center for Health Statistics (NCHS). These are from data collected by the Health Interview Survey, an ongoing nationwide survey based on actual household interviews. Every week a broad range of United States citizens are interviewed by specially trained personnel of the U.S. Bureau of the Census who seek information about a variety of health and other characteristics of each one of us in our civilian and noninstitutionalized population.

The NCHS figures we offer here were obtained from about 42,000 households containing about 134,000 people. The result is a statistically acccurate and ongoing sampling of our population by an experienced staff. The studies cover all four major geographic regions, both urban and rural, all fifty states and the District of Columbia.

Out of all this the NCHS produces its statistical reports, which are dependably comprehensive and detailed. Let's now look at the most recently available figures, most still unpublished but provided to me on special request. I've selected those of greatest significance to the low back problems we're probing in this book. What makes them particularly interesting is that they give a detailed picture of these problems in terms of those involved—their ages, sex, economic status—as well as show clearly how the problem is escalating.

First, however, an explanation of the NCHS term "impairment" because you will find this used often. An impairment in the NCHS' own words is: "a chronic or permanent defect, disabling or not, representing for the most part decrease or

loss of ability to perform functions. . . ." Under this defini-
tion also there is no overlapping; for example, impairment
of back or spine does not include arthritis or disk disease.
Now to the figures.

The epidemic aspects of this problem are quickly made
clear. In 1969 impairments of back or spine (except paralysis) involved 6,500,000 people; in 1971 more than
8,000,000 people suffered such problems. In short, in two
years these problems jumped by nearly a third. Compare this
with a decline during this same period of some 8 percent in
impairments (except paralysis and missing lower extremities)
of the lower extremities and hips.

Let's now look at the frequency of several of these conditions. In 1969 almost 2,000,000 people reported disk problems, and about 20,000,000 suffered with various forms of
arthritis, a very large percentage of which strike the spine as
well or may even involve only the spine. This adds up (disk
problems, plus back or spine impairments) to a definite
10,000,000 suffering back problems, plus perhaps as many
or more arthritics to be added to this total. One might well
speculate that as many as from 20,000,000 to 40,000,000
Americans have back trouble; there are also some
10,000,000 who suffer impairments of "upper extremity and
shoulder" or "lower extremity and hip," some of which are
likely also to fall into the back problems, adding several millions more.

Another measure of the seriousness of back problems is
that impairments of back or spine resulted in nearly
12,000,000 visits to physcians in 1971, and to this again you
must add a sizable number of the 21,000,000 such visits for
arthritis. Many of these patients have also suffered multiple
back operations. Dr. C. Norman Shealy, director of the Pain
Rehabilitation Center of La Crosse, Wisconsin, tells of such
patients whose medical bills ran in one case to $160,000 and
in another to close to $500,000. He reports only recently that
almost 25 percent of all Americans suffer injuries to their
back or spine in their lifetimes, and about 10 percent sustain
actual permanent impairment of their spines.

Some of the material which NCHS has compiled may be of help to you by teaching you the danger sources.

Where Back Injuries Occur

Of the 12,500,000 impairments caused by injuries in the United States in 1971, more than 3,000,000 were of the back and spine, the most frequent injuries of all. Of these, virtually a third occurred at work, a fifth at home, and more than a quarter in a moving vehicle. And in a recent study of industrial injuries, Drs. R. K. Beals and N. W. Hicknan, the University of Oregon Medical School and the Psychology Center, report that 1,250,000 American workers suffer injuries to their backs or spines every year, that more than half of these sustain a permanent disability and that 2,500,000 Americans today have some permanent impairment of the back from an injury.

Those who suffered a back or spine impairment through injury in 1971 were as likely to be male as female, were almost twice as likely to be earning a family income of under $10,000 as over, were only slightly more likely to be employed as not in the labor force; only very few were unemployed. These problems occurred mainly in those between the ages of seventeen and sixty-five.

Knowing the danger areas may help you avoid injury to your back simply by being aware of whether *you* should be more careful. In 1971 the injuries causing impairments to the back or spine were most likely to occur from a moving vehicle (almost 29 percent of these accidents); falls were next in frequency (25 percent), and onetime lifting or exertion did the damage 18 percent of the time.

Why Has All This Become Epidemic?

Just as man developed his low back problems because he crossed nature up and, instead of walking on all fours or clinging to his trees, started to walk about upright, so other changes have produced what is virtually an epidemic of low back pain, discomfort and trouble. The changes are not only in physical behavior but in attitude, family life and personal life-style.

It was well after World War I before anyone would even admit being bothered by backaches, or even admit having them before his or her sixties. That was the day of the stiff upper lip, which would admit of neither complaints nor of physical weaknesses. But life changed in the 1930s, people talked more and expressed emotions more, and with World War II came the "Oh, my aching back!" syndrome. The cry became recognized both as a real and as a growing problem.

Another change has taken place. When Grandpa or old Uncle George would accept the fact that his "lumbago"—his bad back— kept him from working, the large multi-generation family of that era would protect him even though he couldn't work. Instead of throwing him out to seek public charity or starve, the old gentleman would be useful in the large household where he fulfilled tasks such as baby-sitting. He didn't demand more than this and was satisfied to eke out a painful and limited existence in a world where physical limitations were the usual way of life.

Today few men or women would be willing to accept such a half-life. Our intelligence demands that any discomfort be speedily corrected, that "something be done for *that* problem." When there is back pain, it must be corrected with either a pill or surgery or something. And so the doctor sees everyone with more than a passing backache. Since the medical profession is an intimate part of our culture and responds quickly to its pressures, the doctor too looks for active measures to take—offers disk surgery or traction or physiotherapy or one of the new injections. So the figures grow, and backaches seemingly increase—in part because of this cultural change but also in part because there is a real increase in back problems owing to changes in our mode of living.

There's a new vertical mobility that has sharply contributed to the growth of low back problems. People are increasingly stepping out of their roles, and in the course of this they do things they're not accustomed to and set the stage for low back problems. The sedentary clerk goes away on the weekend and plays tennis at an expensive resort, or the heavy laborer tries his hand at skiing or other sports demanding the use of muscles he never uses. Whereas, in earlier times, the sportsman would be a wealthy man who indulged at his club for five or more times a week and so kept in prime athletic shape, everyone is doing it now on the weekend—only everyone isn't in safe shape for it.

The result is an enormous number of strained muscles and backs, slipped disks and whatever. And whereas once people just put up with their suffering as something that had to be endured along with the winter cold and the summer heat, today people insist on having any problem corrected. Few of us are willing today to be has-beens or to accept anything but the highest quality of life. We will go from pillar to post demanding to be restored to top shape.

All these factors have contributed to the epidemic of backaches and the enormous demand for medical care of such problems. Now let's turn to the question of what these low back problems consist of. What is it we're actually talking about, and what does the doctor look for? What are the causes and how can they be diagnosed?

Chapter 4

LOW BACK PROBLEMS:
What You *Must* Tell Your Doctor and
How He Will Examine You

THE SUFFERER who seeks out a doctor for low back problems is considerably different from, say, the one who comes asking help for his headache (another of people's most common ailments). The headache patient, we know, virtually always has the actual source of pain in his head or neck. True, he may have the flu or some other general (systemic) disorder, such as high blood pressure, which originates elsewhere, but the changes that actually produced the headache are in the head itself—such as vascular (blood vessel) changes which take place when one has, for example, the flu or a fever or a hangover. As he may have emotional problems, also arising in the brain.

On the other hand, the person who sees his doctor with complaints of pain in the left arm may be the victim of a heart attack, and the one with pain in the right shoulder blade may well be suffering with a diseased gallbladder. These are instances of referred pain—a condition in which the hurt is felt at a site some distance from the place of the actual disorder.

The low back problem, however, involves a bit of everything. There may be referred pain, a warning of any one of a wide range of conditions elsewhere (stomach ulcers or pancreas disorders or many other difficulties). The low back problem may, for example, produce symptoms without pain (say, weakness or pins and needles or other neurological changes), or it may refer pain down the back of leg, produce

52

sciatica or numbness or paralysis. It may even set off pain right where it starts, in the low back. In short, the low back disorder can be a masquerader, a dissembler, hiding its problems under a variety of symptoms and signs which can give even the knowledgeable doctor a good deal of difficulty in tracking them to their source.

Low back problems cover a wide range of disorders, from those of emotional origin (tension may well express itself in the form of low back pain) to tumors, from muscle strains to spinal fractures, from slipped disks to arthritis, from infections to poor posture. Diagnosis is not always easy, and you can help yourself and your doctor if you come prepared with answers to the questions he is going to ask. Here then is what you should be ready to answer, so think them over while you have the time and can do so.

What You Must Tell Your Doctor

Usually the sufferer is so overwhelmed with the immediate problem, particularly when it's one of severe pain, that it's often hard to get the history needed for a diagnosis. And often, when in pain, the patient forgets certain significant things. Think about all this beforehand, and if necessary, use your family to refresh your memory. After all, they're not in pain and are able to think and remember more objectively and clearly than you can.

It's important to know how the pain or other problem developed. Did it appear suddenly, did it come by itself or following an injury; did it start after you lifted something heavy or only bent forward, perhaps just to pick up a pencil? Think back carefully to whether you had such backaches occasionally or regularly in the past—did long auto trips or heavy lifting, bending or prolonged periods of stooping over cause you low back trouble or whatever it is that's bothering you (say, pain running down the back of your leg or numbness).

Don't be surprised, though, if a knowledgeable physician doesn't seem to accept these reports of how it all started at face value, doesn't immediately label them the cause of your problems, but goes on probing. It's common to find the low back sufferer recalling—with his or her new hindsight—something responsible for the trouble: a fall, say, or lifting a heavy weight.

Lately, I carefully reviewed a group of fourteen patients who came to see me with low back pain and whose problems proved to involve tumors which had spread to their spines. Yet of these, more than a third (five in all) attributed the onset of their problems to an injury. No good physician wants to miss his diagnosis, so your doctor may well go into a long-drawn-out, careful examination with a whole battery of tests when you complain of low back problems.

What to Know About Your Low Back Pain

It's important for you to have noted a series of points and facts about your pain. This may be helpful as a checklist so that you have the proper answers when your doctor asks:
1. Is the pain constant or does it only come intermittently and, if so, at what times during the day or night?
2. Between periods of pain are you completely free of hurt?
3. Where is the pain—in the back or the buttock or the leg or foot—and does it vary in its location?
4. Does the pain awaken you or even keep you from sleeping?
5. Did the pain start suddenly or come on gradually with a steady worsening? (This may warn your doctor of the possibility of a tumor.)
6. Is the pain relieved by bed rest? (This often shows a slipped disk.)
7. Is the pain made worse by standing rather than sitting?
8. Does coughing, sneezing or straining at stool increase the pain?
9. Does forward bending or stooping aggravate the pain?

It's important to be careful in your answers, for only recently one of my medical students wrote on a medical chart that the patient (who was suffering with a severe lumbar disk pain) was not made worse by heavy lifting or stooping. I questioned the patient again, expressing surprise at this reply. He then explained that he just never did any heavy lifting or stooping because of the severe pain.

So be careful with your answers—doctors don't always ask questions the right way. Particularly if they're not highly experienced in a particular area, they may accept a partial answer without probing into what you mean or why you answered as you did. You have to accept some of the responsibility if your answer misleads your physician, and since you will be the one to pay the price, it pays to make certain your doctor understands the exact and entire situation.

Just as it's important to know what aggravates the pain, so it's important to be ready to answer questions relating to the opposite side of the coin, the nonpain:

1. Is the pain relieved when you sit or when you stand?
2. Is there any other particular body position which does relieve the pain?
3. Is there any medication that relieves the pain? (Whether an occasional aspirin or two makes you comfortable or whether you know from experience something more powerful that's needed to stop the pain tells your doctor a good deal about the intensity of the pain and the problem he's dealing with.)
4. What previous treatments have been of help—has heat or cold been more helpful, did low back manipulation relieve the condition or make it worse, did low back supports or girdles help?
5. What was the diagnosis doctors made at a previous episode, or what conditions did they suspect were present?

There are also other symptoms than just pain, and here, too, you must be prepared with certain important facts your doctor will want to know.

The Nonpainful Things to Tell Your Doctor

The spinal column, as you may recall from Chapter 2, carries nerves to and from the brain, brings reports of the sensations in all parts of the body (pain and touch, hot and cold) and takes back orders to the muscles and glands and blood vessels (so that you can walk or stand or salivate or blush). And these sensory and motor nerves come off the spinal cord in paired nerves that slip through spaces in the spinal column.

Let something—anything—press on these nerves, and you suffer pain or distorted sensations or loss of ability to get your orders through properly to your body. So if a slipped disk presses on one of these nerves (there will be a full chapter later on this), it can cause any of these effects, as can a tumor, for it presses mechanically against nerves. In both cases the spinal nerves are trapped by their very defense, the solid bone surrounding them and against which they are squeezed and injured.

We've already considered the things to tell your doctor about the pain that results from low back problems, but here is what you should tell him about the *non*painful symptoms. This will help your physician and yourself; you will get help faster if he knows everything.

Almost everybody today knows that sciatica is a neuralgia of the sciatic nerve (the word comes from the medieval Latin *sciaticus,* or hip joint) which affects the low back, the buttock, the back of the thigh, the calf and often the foot. But although most people think of this as always being pain, the condition may include both pain and other symptoms, or it may encompass just the nonpainful symptoms, which are what we're concerned with right now. Here is a checklist of questions to prepare to answer for your doctor or to inform him on:

1. Have you noticed any numbness or loss of sensation in your back or buttocks, legs or feet? If so, where is it?
2. Have you had any pins-and-needles sensation (what we

call paresthesia) in this same area and, if so, exactly where?

3. Have you had any other odd sensations (hot or cold or whatever) in this area and, again, where?

4. Have you had any difficulties with walking? Does one shoe seem to slap the floor or ground when you walk (you may hear it on a hard surface)? (This is what we call a partial foot drop, a weakness from low back pain or nerve root pressure.)

5. Have you noticed any weakness in a leg, any difficulty in walking on your heels or your toes? (This may show itself in a sudden tendency to trip over small elevations such as a sidewalk curb, a rock or even the edge of a rug. Patients will often first notice this in climbing stairs, often complain that "my leg gives out from under me unexpectedly.")

6. Have you had any increased difficulty in voiding, any constipation recently? Most patients won't think of this, but these changes in bowel and bladder control can and do result from pressure on the spinal cord or its nerve roots.

7. Have you noticed any wasting away, any diminution or emaciation of your thigh or calf, has that of one leg shrunken in comparison to that of the other? (Doctors call this atrophy.)

8. Do you feel any particular change in the way you walk, have you felt any sensations of paralysis? (Patients will tell me, "I'm paralyzed and can't move my legs," but it's only the severe pain that makes it impossible for them to move, and there is no paralysis present.)

Every bit of accurate information you can give your physician will help him—and you—for this isn't always an easy area for the doctor to pin down the problem, and there are many disorders he has to keep in mind when a sufferer comes to him for help.

This may seem obvious, but it's surprising how easy it is for a person who's either in pain or frightened (and everybody is frightened when he or she seeks a doctor's help) to forget or be unable to answer the questions a doctor asks unexpectedly. If you review these at home with a member of the family, proper answers can be framed, things can be recalled by you or someone else in the family, and the whole picture can be made ready for the physician, so he can help give prompt and correct care.

Your Doctor Needs Your History—He Must Know You!

If your physician is to help you, he must know everything about you. Even though I'm called in as a consultant and specialist, I still look to a patient's social history. I want to know what his job is and how he works (is he a perfectionist, does he work under pressure all day long?); what hours he puts in and if he takes his work—and his problems—home with him at nights and on weekends; how he likes or hates his work. I want to know about all his relationships—with his wife, his children, his fellow employees, those under him and those over him. The patient who tries to fool me, to build a favorable picture, is only cheating himself of my best help.

I want to know what he does when he goes home at night (does he stop for a drink?) and what his hobbies are (does he participate in sports or just watch from a soft chair in front of a TV set?). Does he read or go to the movies? I want to know how much he smokes and how much he drinks, if he has a social life and what his sex life is like.

And if he is a she, the questions are the same, depending on what she does. The pattern of questions is the same. I want a good picture of this man or woman whom I'm treating. I want to know him or her as a human being.

Medically, too, I want to know everything—all the diseases patients have ever had and what's bothering them now. What medication do they take, and how often; what have they seen doctors for in the past, and when; and for what have they ever been hospitalized. I want to know what was or what was not found ("The doctor thought my pain might be a heart attack, but everything was normal . . . with all my pain he

wanted to do a thorough checkup, but it was normal . . ."
and so it goes with some).

I want to know about every operation that was performed
and why. It's essential that the physician know if you've had
an operation for, say, breast cancer or prostate cancer, had a
gallbladder removed or been hospitalized for ulcers or had
kidney stones. Every one of these could be the cause of present low back pain, which might be due to referred pain or a
spreading or recurrent cancer, or the pain may have nothing
at all to do with any of these. But it's always important for the
doctor to know, so he can protect you against any of these
possibilities.

The Low Back Examination

The examination for low back dysfunctions may really be
simple because the usual office examination is often entirely
sufficient for a good diagnosis, along with a good and completely accurate history. The complicated affairs like spinal X
rays or blood tests or radioisotopes and the rest (we'll cover
these in detail in the appropriate chapters later) are limited
to the minority of instances where the doctor cannot readily
identify the problem, where he may suspect a tumor or even
advise surgery and want to confirm his suspicions or locate a
slipped disk or a fracture.

In my Low Back Pain Clinic you will probably find much
simpler equipment than your own general practitioner is
likely to have. There are no X ray machines or special gad-
gets for diagnosis. It's strictly a place with a couple of chairs
and an examining table, a rubber hammer or two to test
reflexes and a couple of safety pins for measuring sensation,
a measuring tape to check muscular atrophy.

You just don't need anything very slick or fancy to evaluate the patient with a low back dysfunction. The sophisticated tests such as spinal X rays and radioisotope examinations
are best done in hospitals anyhow, and we don't need them
for the vast majority of sufferers.

Chapter 5

THE PSYCHOLOGY AND MYTHOLOGY
OF LOW BACK PAIN:
What It Is and Isn't

THERE IS a way of talking that human beings use which has become known as organ language. In it we express our feelings or emotions physically: "You make me sick to my stomach. . . . That job gives me a headache. . . . I've got butterflies (or rocks) in my stomach. . . . My heart ached." But probably more than anything else we talk of our backs: "That's a terrible load on my shoulders. . . . My boss is on my tail all the time. . . . I wish my wife would get off my back. . . . We ought to put some backbone in him." Finally, what better way is there to refer to the back than "He ought to stand on his own two legs. He's spineless."

If you notice, all these back references in essence refer to the low back, for this is where the chief strain of carrying any load will go, and this is where the price of learning to walk upright—on our own two legs—has been paid over these hundreds of millions of years. In these organ language expressions—made without thinking and coming out of our deep unconscious feelings—are to be found many of the problems that bother patients and doctors alike, that set off so many of the backaches we see—particularly those of a certain group of these chronic sufferers.

Of course, you must see this in perspective, for there are also very real physical backaches (the slipped disks, the lumbosacral strains, the results of overweight and bad posture, the lack of proper exercise and the like). The purely physical backaches are much more easily coped with by both doctor and patient simply because they yield to proper medical care. On the other hand, the psychogenic (those caused by psychological or emotional factors) backaches either keep recurring when there is some kind of pressure on the sufferer—and these people do suffer—or are constant and even totally disabling.

The importance of this low back pain psychology to *you* lies in the variety of uses to which you can put this information. To be aware of the fact that these patterns are common may alert you to a problem of your own or that of someone close to you. Often just this knowledge may open the way for a sufferer to gain sufficient insight into his problems to control them. It also makes it possible to understand those who do have this problem, for psychogenic backache can be just as painful as any physical disorder, often *is* physical, as we shall see.

Recognizing the fact that there is no reason to be any more ashamed of having a psychogenic backache (most of us do at some time or other) than to have a tension headache, which virtually everybody has at some time in his life, opens the way for the doctor to help you, for he can be frank with you—tell you your backache is functional or nonorganic, the words he's more likely to use than psychogenic. Starting with this, the two of you can then work on your problems, as we shall see.

The Psychiatrist Looks at Low Back Pain

In many patients there is a striking difference between the actual pathology (disease and its physical manifestations) and the amount of low back pain they report (for we can neither see nor measure pain). There just isn't enough pathology in the spine and vertebrae, muscles and nerves to account for their low back pain. It's when this happens that a physician often turns to a psychiatrist for an evaluation, an interview or assessment, so I thought an interview with a leading specialist in this field might give you useful information.

Dr. Pietro Castelnuovo-Tedesco, a professor of psychiatry at the University of California at Los Angeles, is interested in pain problems. He finds he sees more men than women with low back complaints, and frequently these people report some kind of injury at some time to their backs. But since so many of us have had a back injury at some time, he feels that "the question arises why some people are so much more prone to back pain than the rest of the population."

The psychiatrist takes as his starting place the fact that the spine and its supporting muscles have the responsibility of keeping the body erect, that on these structures falls the burden if we carry a heavy weight. And so it is that the carrying of an emotional burden manifests itself through low back pain in some people, those who are likely to use this kind of body language and symbolization.

Dr. Tedesco points out that the psychiatrist called upon to assess a patient with low back pain would look into whether the person was under stress. The psychiatrist would especially want to know whether the person saw himself as carrying burdens beyond his capacity to bear under circumstances where the struggle involved failed to provide the gratifications which were his due or which he felt were. He points out: "One would be particularly on the lookout for burdens experienced physically rather than emotionally; felt as discomfort in the low back, the weight-bearing portions of the body, rather than as psychic burdens. Many people feel in their bodies the discomfort that other people are able to be aware of as emotional discomforts." (A bit like two people who are worried and say, as we all do, "It's a headache"; one recognizes this as anxiety, while the other will actually get a splitting headache.)

These particular low back pain patients are troubled by inner emotional (psychic) struggles over dependency and independence, have difficulties in handling responsibility and job pressures. They are people who feel pressured beyond the point of their natural endurance, feel more put upon than they ought to. Job-related stresses ("the boss is on my back . . . he rides my tail" sort of thing) often express themselves in low back pain. And at home the wife tells the husband to put up the screens on the house; he gets up on the ladder but then develops a backache from being forced to do something he really doesn't feel like doing.

Thus, the job-related or marriage-related stresses often set off backaches in those whom Dr. Tedesco sees as "people who are divided—conscientious and yet rebellious at the same time, can't say no to the boss but really can't say yes either. They say yes, but they protest with their backs. Their problems are simultaneous compliance and rebelliousness, doing and not doing, saying Yes and saying No. They have a reluctance to bear the burdens cheerfully or with enthusiasm."

What Is Pain and How Do We Measure It?

Pain is more than just the physical hurt or the cry of an injured nerve. It's the whole complex emotional reaction that makes the hurt overwhelming (the chest pain that seems to signal a heart attack) or not even noticeable (the child who falls while hurrying to a pile of new toys). Sometimes pains are diagnosed as either physical or emotional, real or imaginary. But to do it this way is to imply a certain judgment which is mistaken. For all pains are "real" to the sufferer—and hurt. The pain of depression is as severe as that of a slipped disk; the "hurt feelings" really do hurt.

What's more, you can't ever fully separate the emotional from the physical, for the physical pain, of necessity, causes an emotional reaction, and the patient who suffers with emotional pain will sooner or later show physical changes in one way or another. The person who suffers with pain—physical or emotional—for six months or more is no longer the person he or she was before it all started.

In short, pain really isn't easily defined, and even if we could define it, it would serve no useful purpose because it's best understood by example and measured by its reaction to treatment. Defining pain is like trying to describe water to someone who has never drunk a glass of it. Doctors tend to judge pain, to measure and evaluate it, by what relieves it; if an aspirin relieves a pain, it's not regarded as being as severe as the pain that requires a morphine injection for relief. We have no pain thermometer, no way we can measure or weigh pain, and this makes it just that much more difficult for you to explain your pain to your physician and for him to understand it.

Then there is another aspect. The acute pains are no problem in medicine today; powerful drugs and anesthetics relieve such problems as lumbosacral strains or permit slipped disk surgery. But the chronic pains are a whole different ball game—Here the doctor has a difficult task because powerful narcotics taken over any extended period of time can—and often do—make addicts of the suffers. And the real problems are those patients who have chronic pain for which there is no apparent organic reason, where any pathology present is minimal and could not be causing such difficulties. But this is a problem by itself.

The Pain-Prone Patient

Dr. George L. Engle, professor of psychiatry at the University of Rochester, introduced the term "pain-prone patient" to characterize a special group of people among whom many chronic low back pain sufferers with no physical causes are commonly found. These people are particularly liable to pain problems of many kinds and have a group of psychological characteristics in varying combinations.

Typically, the parents of such unhappy people—for anyone who suffers pain is unhappy—were punishing and violent individuals who damaged their children with the family atmosphere. The pain-prone patient relieves his or her marked guilt feelings through the pain he or she suffers. And people use their pain as a mode of communication and seek pain through injuries and by operations. They are unable to tolerate success but must suffer. Finally, these unfortunates are very angry and hostile people who cannot express these feelings but instead turn them inward and experience them as pain.

Such people, of course, need a psychiatrist, and the physician must exercise great care in handling them, for they seek out painful and unnecessary examinations and surgery. In fact, Dr. Engle tells of one such man who eventually was relieved of his pain through a series of operations, and as each operation succeeded, new symptoms appeared and psychological deterioration grew. Relief of pain came only with virtually full mental deterioration.

"Doctor, You Must Do Something for This Sufferer!"

This plea has led more doctors into overdoing treatment than is believable. *You* can protect the people you care for by never pressuring doctors in this way—they are only human and may well give in to this plea. One patient I saw as a resident a quarter of a century ago is still vivid in my memory and I hope will always serve to keep me from ever overtreating anyone.

This was a woman who complained of low back and leg pain. A series of special difficult and sometimes irritating spinal X rays were taken and three separate back operations performed. As each one failed, another surgeon was pressured for help until in desperation he agreed to take another look. The original pain increased with each of the spinal examinations and each of the operations. Other procedures to attack main spinal roots were tried, and eventually the patient became paralyzed as a result of all the surgery and procedures, yet the original pain remained undiminished.

At that time prefrontal lobotomies were common, for we had few of the major tranquilizers that are now used with the mentally ill. The woman's brain was attacked and cut (for this is what a lobotomy does), and after major brain surgery her appearance became unsightly. The woman was permanently paralyzed, and despite all this, the original pain was still present.

Whether this was a pain-prone patient or not, I don't know simply because this understanding came nearly a decade after for this unfortunate woman, and we never looked at her in this light. But as I look back now, it would seem more than likely.

The Doctor-Patient Relationship

You can protect yourself against this sort of overtreatment, against the chronic tragedies by being willing to listen openly and without anger if your doctor should tell you that *your* pain is functional, that there's nothing wrong with you. Perhaps you won't believe him, and you might well ask for a consultation if you doubt him (we'll discuss the choice of a doctor or specialist in Chapter 11). If the pain hurts and you are sure it's physical, then you might even seek a second and independent consultation. But if your doctor and your consultant agree, the odds are that they are right.

You will then surely save yourself a lot of grief by accepting their verdict and asking for the help they advise, even if it is psychotherapy. You've already seen what can happen otherwise, and there isn't one of us who is specifically involved in pain who hasn't seen or known of innumerable human beings who've been turned into narcotic addicts or been mutilated by useless surgery in this terrible way. It might help to recall an old folk saying that if three people say you're drunk, you should lie down.

The strongest protection you can have is a good concerned general practitioner who takes ongoing care of you and your family. If you have faith in him, he can help you over many of the humps in life and protect you from a great deal of trouble.

The Myths of Low Back Problems

There is a great deal of mythology—of widespread false beliefs—about the low back and its problems. Scrapping any beliefs you may have in these is the best way to a happier, healthier, more comfortable life. Let's look at these myths and the realities:

1. *First and worst is the belief that if you have low back pain you have to live with it, that it comes with the years and you can't avoid it.* On the contrary, most low back problems can and are treated successfully by doctors—sometimes with as little as simple exercises!

2. *X rays will show the spinal abnormalities, and that's all you need for diagnosis; if there's anything wrong with the low back it can be seen in the X rays.* Actually the X ray findings are frequently untrustworthy in this respect, and your spine just never listens to these myths. We can see X rays of spines so abnormal that we would be prepared to swear the person must be crippled, yet he's in perfect health and comfort. On the other hand, the owner of another and perfectly normal spine—X raywise—can hardly hobble about.

3. *If you have arthritis of the spine, you've "really had it"; you're sure to be all crippled up.* There are many people in old age homes, people whose spines are completely arthritic, who are not bothered by it at all. In fact, many of these people don't even seem to notice anything wrong.

4. *If you have a sore back you should "work it out."* Actually this may well aggravate the condition and totally incapacitate you. You're better off simply resting sore muscles until they're well again.

5. *Heat is always best for the sore back.* Sometimes heat does *not* help, and only cold will. I try one, and if it doesn't help, I try the other.

6. *Heavy laborers are the likely victims of lumbosacral strains and slipped disks, not desk jockeys.* Some people can be

stevedores all their lives and never have back problems, while the white-collar worker may bend down to pick up a piece of paper and suffer a lumbosacral strain or a slipped disk.

7. *Taking off excess weight will automatically rid you of your back pain.* Excess weight is certainly bad for your back, but some people take off weight and still have low back pain, and we don't know why.

Part II

*The Special Low Back Problems
and Their Help*

Chapter 6

SEX, YOU AND THE
LOW BACK PROBLEMS

SEX AND backaches have long been the butt of innumerable jokes, but there *is* a very real connection between sex, your own sex and your low back problems (your likelihood of getting them and even which ones). The involvement of sex in low back pain is very considerable, and both sexes are entangled in it, although the classic jokes do tend to be strongly one-sided. Typical is the story of the couple who were walking in the zoo when a gorilla seized the wife and carried her off for some quick sex. The wife called out to her husband, "What shall I do?" He thought for a moment; then his face suddenly brightened. "Tell him about your backaches."

Out of this sort of thing with its basis in reality has come the remark that the world's greatest contraceptive is the backache. What is overlooked, however, is that there is also a category of men who will use any excuse to explain their own lack of sexual prowess, and to them, too, the low back pain becomes a useful excuse. This is very common in industrial accidents. "I can't have sex anymore since I slipped and fell, hurting my back" is invariably thrown in during compensation hearings. Although I suspect this complaint has some validity, it's difficult to determine just how much. Where money is involved, there is a tendency to throw in everything—and how can you prove the claimant is lying here?

However, it is interesting to note that what was once a sexually oriented cause of low back problems in woman has now become increasingly a problem for men as well.

High Heels and the Low Back

The most common low back problem that patients and doctors alike have to contend with is the chronic lumbosacral strain (much of Chapter 8 will be devoted to it). Typically this shows itself in a combination of low back pain and fatigue and mostly in women, with the bulk of victims past the age of thirty-five. However, I would anticipate the possibility of now seeing the condition spreading more to men—not because they're changing their sex but simply because the fashions have markedly changed. For high heels play a definite role in this problem, and men are now turning to these as the latest fad. When you wear an elevated or high heel, it puts your foot on a sort of slant. It's just as if you were standing on the side of a sharply sloping hill and facing down toward the bottom, the valley below. If you can imagine or already know the feeling of wearing high heels, you will realize that you don't lean forward despite the fact that the shoe is built so that this would happen were it not for your built-in stabilizers; your body automatically compensates for this forward pitch. You correct this strange angle by leaning backward and so increase the natural curvature of your low back (the lumbar lordosis), and you also swivel your hips a bit. In short, you become swaybacked (increasing the lumbar lordosis), which is definitely *not* good for your back.

Earth Shoes and Your Low Back

According to the New York *Times* recently, Earth shoes came out of Denmark, originally designed and built by a former couturier and a student of yoga who insisted on astrologically checking the birth dates of an American couple before she finally permitted them to market her shoes here. Even then the shoes were to be sold only on a side street and not advertised. The idea was that people should have to discover them by themselves, and they did, starting with college students about four years ago. However, 10 percent of those who try them out are said to be unhappy with them and can't wear them at all. Just one last note before we talk about what the shoes do—the people who sell the shoes are usually young, and one fringe benefit offered any six-month employee is a course in Transcendental Meditation for which the shoe company foots the bill.

The usual women's shoes and now, increasingly, men's as well have low soles and high heels (even the platform shoes have relatively high heels, compared to the soles). But the Earth shoe has a high sole and a low heel. In short, it does just the opposite of what high-heeled shoes do; instead of throwing you forward, it literally sets you back on your heels. Instead of increasing your lumbar lordosis, it flattens it out.

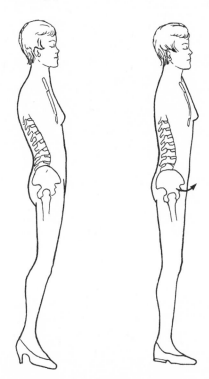

Figure 6. Wearing high heels results in a compensatory increase in lumbar lordosis.

You'll surely hear a considerable number of testimonials from people saying, "I've had back pain, but when I started to wear those Earth shoes, it all cleared up." Looking at it medically, we must admit that one of the factors involved in chronic backaches is an increased or exaggerated lumbar lordosis, the individual with the swayback. Such an individual may well be improved by wearing this new type of shoe (there are a whole bunch of takeoffs on the original concept, and other companies are getting into the act now).

So the Earth shoe has its value—but only in certain people. It's *not* a cure-all, and it's not going to take every person with back trouble and make him better. There will be no benefit for the sufferer with a slipped disk which is causing pressure, and there's a whole range of problems which won't be helped. Let me emphasize: *There's no one approach, no one form of treatment, no basic philosophy that's going to answer all low back pain problems!* I just can't seem to repeat this often enough for both doctors and patients.

Pregnancy and Low Back Pain

There are really two problems here: women who had low back problems before they became pregnant and so started off with a problem which can only be worsened by the pregnancy, and those who have never had any back difficulties before. In either case, some degree of low back pain is the rule during the last two or three months of pregnancy.

This pain usually consists of a dull, aching sensation involving the entire low back and is usually aggravated by prolonged standing, walking or climbing stairs. If you should be troubled by this sort of problem, you will find it can usually be relieved by either sitting down or—more effectively—by lying down. However, bending backward or leaning forward (extension or flexion of your back) will make the pain worse. Sometimes one of the corsets designed to provide the pregnant woman with low back support will help.

However, these are only stopgap measures intended to get

you over a forty- or fifty-day period, for the majority of women even with severe pain during the last three months will be relieved of their pain once the delivery is over and they are able once more to go about their usual activities. The vast majority of pregnant women who suffer with low back pain are made fairly comfortable with a program of reduced physical activities, mild painkillers (analgesics) and a supporting corset although sometimes the pain is so bad that prolonged bed rest is necessary.

However, sometimes those who have already had two or more children find the problem can reach a severity where rest is not enough. Here the use of a contraption which almost resembles something from the Spanish Inquisition may be used. From a frame hanging over the bed a series of straps connect to a canvas sling supporting the woman's entire pelvic area; traction weights may also be attached. The sufferer is kept in this for a couple of weeks, followed by her wearing a canvas pelvic support for several months.

The pain is believed caused by a softening or relaxation of the ligaments involving the pelvis and the lumbar spine. This may even include the annulus of the lower spinal disks, and if there is any preexisting weakness, there may be a severe herniated or slipped disk with all the problems that introduces. During pregnancy only conservative measures such as bed rest or traction and medication are used. Surgery is reserved for those rare instances when the slipped disk proves so damaging that it causes paralysis with loss of sensation and even involvement of bladder and bowel functions through pressure on the nerves to those organs' sphincters.

I've seen a considerable number of women who date the onset of all their low back difficulties to an earlier pregnancy. We don't really know just why this happens, but I suspect it may be due to the softening of the pelvic and lower lumbar ligaments which never again improve to their prepregnant conditions but instead leave a persistent low back problem. To recover from these effects of your pregnancy, you should follow the exercises your doctor can prescribe for you.

These, in fact, are not very different from those we'll describe in Chapter 15.

Low Back Pain During the Menstrual Period: Surgery?

Studies both here and abroad seem to show that the backaches experienced during the menstrual period are not connected with any emotional or psychological problems, as has sometimes been said, but are physical or physiological in nature. In general, gynecologists use mild analgesics usually successfully to control this problem.

When there are severe intractable pain problems associated with menstruation, gynecologists have even performed hysterectomies. But this has only a spotty record of success, and the whole idea is defended by some and attacked by others. It is widely conceded that a good many unnecessary hysterectomies are being performed so that such an operation should be regarded with a good measure of skepticism, and its need should be checked with other doctors before you agree to so radical and little-proved a procedure for menstrual pain. Every possible alternative should be explored before you even think of a hysterectomy for menstrual pain, however severe.

Male Chauvinist Backache

It has a jawbreaking name—ankylosing spondylitis—but it's also known as Marie-Strumpell disease and even bamboo spine. It starts with low back pain, and nine out of ten of its victims are men. It usually begins in the teens or the twenties, and its onset is relatively uncommon after thirty years of age. It's a progressive condition in which the spinal ligaments and the vertebral column with its disks become ossified, hardening like bone. The victims have a limited degree of chest expansion in breathing and develop a typically hunchbacked or stooped kind of appearance with a stiff, hardened spine. Since it first strikes the low back and sacroiliac joints, the pain starts there and in the legs, but it takes ten to twenty years for the condition to develop fully. We will talk more of this in Chapter 10, for this is a strange form of the arthritic disorders.

Other Male Low Back Problems

Where the low back is concerned, men on the whole would seem to have a bad time. Lumbosacral strain—the worst pain you can have in the low back—can occur at any age but occurs most often between the ages of twenty-five and fifty, striking men twice as often as women. The pain, which often covers a wide area, starts as a stiffness that traps the patient into the belief it's not so bad and he can work it off—only he ends up by being carried into the hospital on a stretcher. The pain is so unbelievably bad that even the gentlest handling of the stretcher causes terrible agony. Yet the condition is readily treated, and recovery is prompt and dramatic. But the condition is so complex and common that the details are best left for their own chapter (8, to be specific).

The slipped disk (disk disease, herniated disk, all the same disorder) is another condition that strikes men more often than women—three times as often to be exact. Actually slipped disks are extremely common. Most patients past thirty-five reveal X ray evidence of this condition, and most are symptom-free, yet this is the most feared of all spinal disorders. Again we have a very complex condition which is best reserved for a chapter (9) all its own.

Sex and the Low Back Problems

Certainly any marked degree of pain is going to destroy all sexual desire, but some problems are more closely connected with sexual difficulties than others, and low back pain is one of these. The jokes we spoke of at the beginning of this chapter are simply indicative of the widespread recognition of this fact. Dr. Beverley T. Mead, professor of psychiatry at

Omaha's Creighton University, recently pointed out that backaches are one of the good examples of those common women's complaints which carry strong sexual connotations. The psychiatrist points out that a persistent backache in a woman may be an expression of her fears of becoming pregnant or of her wish to avoid sex. Like headaches, her backaches may be her symbolic way of protesting against sexual activity or her defense against the act itself.

But sometimes sex and the low back become tied together in a straightforward physical way. There is, for example, a condition known as a sacral nerve root cyst (the cyst is a sac filled with fluid) which often must be removed because it presses on the sacral nerves and produces the same effect as a slipped disk. However, when the cyst is removed, it may cause a loss of sensation over the whole area which the nerve supplies, and this numbness may extend over part of the penis, resulting in a serious impairment of sexual function. Other spinal surgery, too, may cause damage to certain of the nerves in this general area so that most men in these rare situations will report a significant degree of sexual impotence and even failure to ejaculate after surgery.

Chapter 7

THE DIFFERENT AGES OF MAN AND THEIR LOW BACK PROBLEMS

WE'VE ALREADY seen how the spine alters with age—how the simple C curve of the fetus becomes the increasingly complex and vaguely S-shaped curve of the child of two. These changes go on into adulthood as the original thirty-three vertebrae gradually develop and fuse so that the adult ends up with only twenty-six separate vertebrae through the union of the original five sacral vertebrae into a single bone, the sacrum, and as the four coccygeal ones fuse into a single coccyx. Along with this, everything else changes with age— the muscles, the tendons and ligaments, the intervertebral disks, the bone of the spine. Even the pattern of low back problems themselves are age-dependent.

Take, for example, a personal experience of my own. I was in my mid-forties when I decided to try sport parachute jumping for the first time. The teaching school supplied the parachutes from their supply of various sizes. When it came my turn, I could hear the parachute jump master call out to the supply room, "Give him the large parachute—he's over forty-five." These people certainly didn't know anything about the physiology of bone or the ways in which that tissue changes, yet they knew from experience that one of the dangers at this age was the likelihood of a compression fracture of the spine.

When you reach the mid-forties, your bones are a little low on calcium so that trauma which could be safely endured by a younger person might produce a compression or a wedge fracture. This is called wedge because the vertebral body can be seen in an X ray to look wedge-shaped rather than the normally block or rectangular shape. By using a larger parachute, you land with a little less impact; you hit the ground more gently and with a softer bounce. This is important even in the aging person who doesn't suffer from senile osteoporosis, for the older bone normally cannot tolerate the jolt that a younger bone can take in stride.

Because the susceptibility to low back problems increases as we get older for a variety of reasons, there are precautions to be taken, awareness of the effects of aging that are essential to the full life. With a slightly changing life-style and a different approach to bodily care, these difficulties can be avoided.

The Child and the Teenager

This is a period where back problems are at an absolute minimum, but they are not entirely absent. So few are the occurrences of arthritis and disk disease at this age that the National Center for Health Statistics (NCHS) finds that the figures for these problems are not sufficiently numerous to offer enough reliability to allow them to calculate how many occur in each 1,000 persons. I would guess that about 1 in every 100,000 patients with a slipped disk is a child under the age of twelve, and we're just not sure why these rare few do occur. While this is certainly more common in the teenager, it's still a rarity during adolescence.

However, youngsters do get disk infections, and this can be a devastating condition, starting with sudden fever and low back pain, along with a feeling of general discomfort or of being just plain out-of-sorts. One three-year-old bent down to pick up a toy, then couldn't straighten up. She had excruciating pain, which was aggravated by any movement of her back or legs, but nothing wrong could be found. An exhaustive medical in-hospital study revealed only a slight change in the sedimentation rate of the blood (it settled faster than normal, a mild indication of something wrong, a change often occurring in infections).

With bed rest the child's pain eased, and the sedimentation rate slowly returned to normal, although the back muscles remained in spasm and the usual curvature children have in the small of their back was flattened out. Because the initial lumbar spine X rays taken shortly after admission to the hospital were normal, after four weeks in the hospital she was sent home with a vague diagnosis of a vertebral inflammation (spondylitis) of unknown origin. It was not until six weeks later (when the acute symptoms had eased) that follow-up X rays revealed clear evidence of a disk space infection.

This sort of thing is typical of this strange condition in children under five years of age. They get a disk infection from an unknown source, probably because in young children there are tiny blood vessels running into the disks, and these can carry infecting bacteria (these vessels normally disappear from the disks by the end of the teens). In these young children this infection is usually due to "staph" (staphylococcus) and first shows itself in a refusal to walk, followed by back pain, stiffness, irritability and fever, along with a lack of appetite and a loss of weight. The whole affair usually lasts less than three weeks and is treated with antibiotics.

In very young children disk infection usually clears up without doing any damage, whereas in older children and teenagers the disease tends to follow more the pattern of adult infection with destruction of the vertebrae. You will find more on this in Chapter 10, but here it might be helpful to consider the various problem areas (muscles, tendons, ligaments, the vertebrae and the disks) and follow the changes that take place in the person with time—along with some tips on protection and care and ways to prevent damage.

Low Back Muscles, Ligaments and Tendons: Time Changes and Protection

The greatest protection for the human back is having strong, supple, elastic muscles, tendons and ligaments. Every athlete—knowing nothing about neurosurgery or orthopedics or physiology—is aware of this, and you see its proof every time you watch a physical contact sport on TV. Just look at how the football or basketball players bend and twist and perform all sorts of stretching exercises to warm up before they enter the game. This is to increase the suppleness and elasticity of their muscles, ligaments and tendons so that these tissues won't be stiff or contracted when they start using them violently. It's this suppleness and elasticity which prevents damage or injuries to their backs.

The professional athlete, of course, is a superb physical specimen. He has come through years of testing by combat. Anyone with weaknesses has long since been weeded out. As a result, you don't see very much in the way of low back injuries or problems among professional athletes.

But where the sports take their toll is in those like one thirty-year-old patient who came to me with complaints of low back pain. Here was a young man beginning to feel the effects of time even at his young age simply because he was trying to do too much. He worked in a factory and was perfectly comfortable during the day except for his lunch break, at which time he played basketball for an hour or so. He was actively engaged in this sport, played on a team several times a week and indulged in a lot of practicing as well.

His muscular activity was simply too strenuous for the nonprofessional competitive athlete of his age. His inherent weaknesses were being brought out by a combination of age changes (these start as we pass through the twenties, which is why even professional athletes are often regarded as old by thirty-five) and what for my patient was overactivity. I hate to change anyone's life-style, to take any pleasure away, but the only prescription possible here was to give up strongly competitive physical contact sports.

Coming back now to the ligaments and tendons—these are strong glistening white sheets of fibrous tissue, alike except in their tasks. The tendons attach the muscles to the bones, while the ligaments hold the joints together. The spine has ligaments running its full length, as well as short ones, and this complicated system was explained in Chapter 2. If you were to examine the tissues of muscles, tendons and ligaments under the microscope, you would see a combination of elastic fibers and nonelastic fibrous tissue.

Under the microscope you can clearly tell the difference between young and old tendons, muscles and ligaments. In the young tissues the proportion of elastic fibers to the nonelastic tissue is clearly much higher than in the old, where nonstretching fibrous tissue gradually becomes predominant over the years from twenty to sixty-five.

Suppleness is the hallmark of youth. This is why my teenage son could, without a warm-up even at the beginning of the season, go out and play several hours of tennis with only moderate stiffness. Later his slight discomfort would quickly pass without ill effects. On the other hand, if I were to do such a thing without slowly building up to this point over a period of time, my low back couldn't take it, and I might be crippled for days, even land in the hospital.

To protect your muscles, ligaments and tendons, a warm-up is essential before any game, particularly if it's a rough contact sport. This makes the tissues supple and protects them and your back. The amount of warm-up is dependent on three things: your athletic condition (how often and regularly you play the game); how long it has been since you played regularly (is it an everyday exercise for you or the season's first?); and how old you are.

If you indulge in sports or exercise regularly (a daily swim, long walks or bicycling), your muscles and the other tissues will always be supple and elastic so your warm-up can be minimal, particularly if you play that particular game every day. But your age is the vital factor. Regular exercise can keep tissue supple and elastic, but an old tendon is still an old tendon, and while you can make the most of the elastic fibers there, no amount of activity is going to make it young again, to increase the elastic tissue.

The old adult (say, the over sixty-five) has to allow himself three or four times as much in warm-up as the young adult in his twenties or thirties—say, forty or fifty minutes or more, compared to fifteen. The older adult should build up gradually at the beginning of the season—perhaps just going out on the tennis court and swinging the racket, hitting just a few balls back and forth the first time.

How the Spinal Disks Age

Your disk starts out with a lot more gellike center (the nucleus) than it will end up with. It also loses its water content. In fact, your height will decrease from when you are thirty-five years old until you pass sixty simply because of these alterations in your spinal disks, and these changes can cost you as much as a half-inch from your overall height.

The result can be seen thus: The older disk is a little flatter, less squishy, more firm, less resilient, more fibrous than the younger one, which is more resilient. Experiments have shown that the young-adult disk will yield and deform only at pressures exceeding 1,400 pounds, while it will take only about 350 pounds to do the same thing to the disks of an older individual. These experiments were carried out on isolated spinal segments of fresh human cadavers (commonly two vertebrae and the disk between them were used).

What this means in practical terms is that by the time you reach forty and move on in life you are certain to lose some of the mobility of your back, which owes its flexibility to the disks and which they alone can provide (the bones obviously can't). Again, as with the soft tissues, no matter how active you may be, no matter how much you keep in shape, there is still a decreased mobility in an old back compared to a young one. Finally, the bones as well undergo changes with the passage of time.

Time and the Spinal Bones

Your bones too get softer with age, and like the changes in disks this is a matter of a steady lifetime change, beginning almost with birth and continuing into very old age. Young bones have more calcium than older ones; they look whiter in X rays and are tougher. It has been shown that the lumbar spine's resistance to pressure in its long axis drops by some 20 percent every decade after the age of thirty so that whereas the vertebral body of a young adult can take as much as 1,000 to 1,300 pounds, that of the elderly may fail after only 300.

This loss of calcium is called decalcification as it goes on gradually, but it may continue in many to the point where it merges over into the area we call pathology or disease and then it becomes senile osteoporosis.

Senile Osteoporosis

Senile osteoporosis is actually a lifetime process which is extremely common. It starts in the forties and becomes significant only when you reach old age. In this condition there are no symptoms, and the condition is discovered only if someone takes an X ray for some other reason or there is a fracture of a bone (commonly the spine) owing to the developing weakness and not to the trauma or injury which is often very minor. It's a strange and little understood condition with racial overtones and certain problems all its own which are best left to Chapter 8.

Protecting the Middle-Aged and Older Back

To accomplish this, you must accept the need to *think defensively* right from the start. You must start preparing in youth for middle age and then for old age. You must recognize that changes come on gradually, and you can work with them but can't fight them. You must recognize that if you're going to let yourself go and not exercise, not be in optimum condition, it's just bound to interfere with your life. I'm not talking of gross obesity here, but even that little bit of a pot and the slight loss of resilience in your younger years.

With the changes we've discussed it's obvious that you're

more vulnerable to low back dysfunction in your later years. But if you keep your muscles in good condition either with regular sports or with planned exercises such as we detail in Chapter 19, this will maintain the maximum suppleness and elasticity of the low back tissues—and a healthier and more comfortable back. But you do have to be consistent. If you want to spend your spare time sitting, watching TV or reading, fine, but then accept the fact that you'll be much more limited in anything you do than your neighbor who swims or bicycles or walks an hour or two every day. And never try to do what he does—whether shoveling snow or swimming or doing repairs around the house.

Living Defensively with Old Age

This is the key to a comfortable aged back. You've got to take a long hard look at yourself, add up the present and the past and make sure you don't try to go beyond them.

We all must face the fact that the older man is not as strong as the younger man, for as you age, you lose some of your muscle, and you can't do the things you did years before. It's easy to see the difference in build: The younger man is wider in the shoulder and narrower in the waist, while the older man tends to get narrower in the shoulder and bigger in the waist.

If an older person has been athletic all his life and has indulged in a sport often and regularly throughout the years, he certainly should keep it up within reason. You can't play football at eighty, but men do play tennis at that age. But when you're older, it's no longer possible or safe to be an occasional athlete. You can't sit around the house all winter and then suddenly in the summer go out and play a fast tennis game. If you want to indulge in any activity, make sure you do it often enough—or don't do it at all.

If you want to start a new sport late in life, it might be wise to discuss it first with your doctor, start slowly and build up to it, then do it often. A good rule of thumb is that when you play a sport, you shouldn't suffer afterward. If after swimming or tennis or whatever you need aspirin and a hot tub and still don't get over the effects for several days, either forget the sport or start doing it often enough so that there is nothing but slight soreness for a half day or so afterward. *Think defensively,* and your back will take care of itself for you.

Even more dangerous on the whole than sports is the house itself. The same man who wouldn't think of endangering his back on the tennis court will start moving furniture around by himself—and end up with a slipped disk or a lumbosacral strain. Or he'll go out—after spending years with no more exercise than padding back and forth between the kitchen and the TV set with a dish of peanuts—and start shoveling snow or try to repair something on the floor and remain stooped over for an hour or two while working.

Middle-aged and older women are much more sensible in this respect than men; they usually call a man to do the heavy lifting or moving of furniture or whatever. Besides, the women are usually in better shape anyhow because they have never retired. They keep scrubbing and cleaning, climbing stairs or shopping as long as they live. And housework is really good, vigorous exercise.

Chapter 8

OSTEOPOROSIS AND LUMBOSACRAL STRAIN: One of People's Worst Pains

THESE TWO disorders are alike in that one is the most common low back problem physicians see in their practice, while the other affects virtually all of us sooner or later. Yet these two are also opposites. Typically they strike people at the different ends of the life span; one is more common among women while the other occurs much more often among men; one is often overwhelming in its paralyzing pain, whereas the other is almost a disease without a symptom; one can be made to disappear as quickly as it struck, leaving no physical damage afterward, while the other leaves a trail of weakness behind it; for one the majority of all doctors know and use almost the same treatment all over the world, but for the other disorder, doctors use widely differing treatments, some of which are very new and promising.

If I see a patient wheeled into the hospital on a stretcher and in such pain that as little as leaning against the litter produces agonies of pain, if the man is afraid of even blinking his eyes for fear of the pain, I'm likely to suspect an acute lumbosacral strain. Certainly this condition can cause the worst and most agonizing of the low back pains, and this includes even the more commonly feared slipped disk.

On the other hand, there was the woman about seventy years old who came to see me with severe back pain and tenderness in her low back. Somewhat hunchbacked and rather short, she had stepped off an unexpected curb and came down hard on her heel. This slightly jarring shock abruptly changed the usual dull, vague ache she'd had for some years to a sharp, severe hurt, which continued unremittingly. Even before I examined the spinal X rays I had taken, I knew with a fair degree of certainty that she had fractured a vertebra and probably had generalized osteoporosis.

Unfortunately, recognizing these two conditions isn't always this simple, for they are often neither so obvious nor so typical. Let's now look into both these very widespread problems and learn something about the disorders themselves, how and why they occur and how we go about treating them.

Osteoporosis and the Low Back

Osteoporosis is just what the name says—a porosity of the bone (the word comes from the Greek *osteon,* meaning bone). The bone in this condition doesn't change in its volume; it loses its density. To understand this, you must know something about this important tissue (for bone itself is actually osseous tissue, the hardest of the connective tissues, which includes cartilage, ligaments and tendons).

Basically, bone consists of a protein matrix which acts as a framework in which calcium salts (chiefly calcium phosphate and calcium carbonate) are deposited to produce the hard substance known as bone. In a way, this is not unlike the construction of a cement floor of a building: Here a metal wire mesh is laid down, and into this is poured the cement which will give hardness and rigidity to the framework, thus producing the floor. But in bone the protein matrix acts not only as a framework, but also as the site for the deposition of calcium, which cannot be laid down if that matrix is missing.

Bone is also a unique living tissue in that it is constantly in a state of flux. Throughout life, bone is continuously being absorbed and remodeled and laid down anew to adjust to the constantly changing pressures, uses and demands of everyday life. It's even been said that every bone in your body is completely absorbed and rebuilt at least once every seven years or so. Sometimes, however, something interferes with this normal replacement, and that's when you get osteoporosis; the absorption of the bone goes on while the formation, the replacement, is reduced.

THE CAUSES OF OSTEOPOROSIS

This disorder may arise from an absorption of the bone matrix with poor replacement, a destruction of the bone matrix or an inadequate production of the matrix.

The majority of the instances of osteoporosis we see are postmenopausal or senile types, and while we have clues and suspicions as to the causes, none of these has yet been fully proved. It's even uncertain whether this is a normal physiological or pathological process of aging. Deficiencies of sex hormones, calcium, phosphate and protein; chronic acidity and overproduction of heparin (a complex anticoagulant principal found in many tissues, especially liver and lung); and even a deficiency of growth hormone all have come under suspicion, but none has been entirely accepted as the real villain. A calcium deficiency, for example, does produce osteoporosis in certain animals, but its role in man is still unproved.

There *are* some known causes for osteoporosis in human beings, but these are responsible for only a minority of the cases we see:

1. Very serious lack of protein, calcium and vitamin C for long periods (such as occurs in starvation or extreme dietary fads).
2. Long-standing immobilization such as occurs with plaster casts in severe fractures or with paralyzed limbs.
3. Prolonged periods of weightlessness (the hope is that programmed exercises during prolonged space voyages will control this).
4. Large doses of corticosteroids (such as cortisone) for long periods of time.
5. Certain endocrine diseases such as acromegaly.

6. Some genetic abnormalities such as mongolism.
7. Pregnancy—but only very rarely.

WHO OSTEOPOROSIS STRIKES: WHEN, WHERE AND HOW

Senile or postmenopausal osteoporosis is a disease that takes a lifetime to develop, and it involves the entire population to some extent. It starts in the mid-thirties, but the loss of bone density doesn't really become significant until old age. It's been estimated that there are 4,500,000 to 5,000,000 postmenopausal women in the United States with this condition.

Osteoporosis may affect the entire skeleton, but it seems to strike the spine in particular and is often identified radiographically (by X ray) only in the vertebral column. It may attack here especially because the vertebrae have an abundant blood supply and are an active blood-forming center of the body. This situation could be expected to induce a quicker response to any increased bodily demands for calcium, draining such bones first of their calcium.

Microscopic measurements of the hipbone (the iliac crest) show a normal loss in the amount of bone with age. In fact, there's a 40 percent drop occurring between the ages of twenty and eighty, with the soft center of the bones showing an equal loss for men and women. But if the hard outer layer of bone is measured, the rate of bone loss is definitely greater in women.

Osteoporosis is clearly more common in women. There are racial differences as well: The disorder occurs much more often in Caucasians than in the other races, but in Israel it is seemingly more frequent in the European Jewish than the Asian. Some people have attributed these differences to the less strenuous physical activities of the Caucasians. But I believe this may be in considerable part due to the same sort of thing that happens when a rich man and a poor man start spending money at the same time and rate—the rich man will still be rich after twenty years, while the poor man will long have run out of funds and got into serious trouble. While the Caucasian is having serious problems, blacks, for example, have sturdier bones to start with, and even though they lose calcium at the same rate as whites they will be more likely to have enough left to prevent trouble when they get old.

THE SYMPTOMS OF OSTEOPOROSIS AND THE PRICE

In many cases this is a disease without symptoms, but even in these instances there is always the high risk of spinal fractures with all the serious problems this occurrence involves.

Osteoporosis does carry with it a high incidence of low back pain, for it particularly affects the weight-bearing vertebrae. The loss of bone density in this condition doesn't always parallel the symptoms, and periods of discomfort are often interspersed with long pain-free periods. The pain is probably due to the pressure of fractured bone on either spinal nerve roots or sensory nerve fibers in the tissues covering the vertebrae. Although many times the pain is present before X rays show a fracture, this is probably because there are microscopic fractures which don't show on X rays.

This condition can be present for years without symptoms until some very minor trauma causes the decalcified vertebra to collapse. Coughing, turning in bed, stepping off a curb or into a depression or a rut in the street, bending forward to pick up a pencil all can cause this vertebral collapse—or there may be no known trauma. The victim may have a kyphosis (from the Greek *kyphos,* meaning bent or hunchbacked) or humpback (the "dowager's hump") and there may be an unexpected reduction in height (as much as five inches) or a back muscle spasm. With these more serious effects the low back pain may be severe.

OSTEOPOROSIS: TREATMENT AND PREVENTION

Osteoporosis is a hard disease to treat, and the best approach is prevention. Tragically, osteoporosis is still virtually a disease without a cure. We have tried both male and female sex hormones, but while these make the victims feel better, they seem to offer no material long-term advantages. Sodium flouride, too, has been tried in the hope that it would stimulate bone formation, and it has been tried in combination with vitamin D and calcium, but the results have been disappointing. It will be twenty years before we know, for example, whether the fluoridation of water supplies prevents this condition because the disease takes so long to develop that those who drink this fluoride must have time to develop the condition before we can tell whether this treatment really works.

It is important to have a high-protein diet so sufferers will maintain an adequate general nutritional condition. Increased activity, too, is important in that it stirs up bone-forming activity. So the best management may well be prophylactic with adequate calcium intake (your doctor can judge this for you) and adequate physical activities in your early and middle years.

Only recently a Mayo Clinic team has introduced an investigational treatment which gives these people a combination of sodium fluoride, oral calcium and vitamin D along with estrogen (a female sex hormone), and this looks promising, but it's a long way from proved. In fact, even its safety is not yet fully established.

The Miseries of Lumbosacral Strain: Acute and Chronic

Lumbosacral strain is the label (we call it diagnosis) physicians use more frequently than any other when low back dysfunctions are brought to them for help. Yet despite the fact that this is the most common low back problem we see in medical practice today, knowledge of it is considerably less than that of many of the other and less frequently seen low back disorders that also cause suffering. It's really an ambiguous sort of condition which can't be proved through X rays or laboratory tests. As a result, when a doctor sees some harmless low back pathology or X ray abnormality, he usually prefers to blame these as the cause of the pain simply because he's trained to look for "hard" proof in his diagnosis, something he can see or feel.

Wastebasket Diagnosis?

The dramatic appearance of some lumbosacral strains—like the one with which we began this chapter—makes these occurrences easy to diagnose, but they are the exception in this widespread problem. Many conditions first labeled as lumbosacral strains later prove—as the true condition gradually develops into a more easily diagnosable entity—to be other problems (early stages of slipped disks, for example).

Since our knowledge of the lumbosacral strain is limited and there is no clear-cut X ray or laboratory evidence that we can yet use, there is some tendency to regard this strain as a wastebasket diagnosis into which is thrown everything a doctor isn't sure of in the way of low back problems. But this should not be so, for lumbosacral strain is a very specific condition with distinct characteristics and two different types—the acute and the chronic.

LUMBOSACRAL STRAIN: FACT VS. FICTION

The facts we do know about this condition are often at variance with some of the beliefs. It can occur at nearly any age, but it's most common during the active years, from twenty-five to fifty, and about two out of every three patients stricken with it are men. Yet statistics prove that the heavy laborer is more liable to lumbosacral strain than is the sedentary worker. Nor is any particular physique or body build any more susceptible than any other—with the single exception of the grossly obese people whose weight is clearly connected to their increased incidence of this low back problem.

However, should the fat person reduce his excess weight,

his lumbosacral strain pain will often persist. And while unequal leg lengths are often found in people who have never had this condition or any other low back dysfunction, such a person who does suffer with lumbosacral strain can often find help by using heel lifts which correct his leg length difference. Clearly we're not dealing with any simple problem, so let us look further into the two kinds.

THE CHRONIC LUMBOSACRAL STRAIN

This is essentially a disease of mechanical stress on the lower spine and is due to a combination of bad posture and inadequate muscles which occurs so often among Americans that this condition has become the most common low back problem seen by many doctors. It's most likely to affect those past the age of thirty-five, a time at which the spinal ligaments begin to lose their elasticity and suppleness, becoming more fibrous and stiff. Before this age the elastic spinal ligaments can still compensate for the excessive demands put on the low back by poor posture and inadequate musculature.

The most serious danger in the chronic lumbosacral strain is that if it lasts for enough years, it will eventually produce degenerative changes in the vertebrae along with osteoarthritis (see Chapter 10). These changes in turn produce additional mechanical low back dysfunction and make the handling of the whole matter more complicated and more difficult.

Most of these sufferers complain of an aching discomfort in their low back. This ache usually covers a wide area rather than a specific spot, and victims usually describe their problem as "fairly severe" or even "mild," only rarely as "very severe." The trouble has usually been present for a long time, and the patients can't be too specific about when it started. Even when there is some remembrance of a fall or injury, careful questioning usually uncovers the fact that the discomfort actually preceded the trauma.

Next to their pain, chronic lumbosacral strain victims complain most often of fatigue, which they feel even when they get enough sleep. Their pain often appears during times of general fatigue, and many complain of a "tired feeling in the back" rather than actual hurt. Almost any activity makes the pain worse, and bed rest usually relieves it.

CHRONIC LUMBOSACRAL STRAIN: WHAT THE SUFFERER IS LIKE

I can't recall seeing this problem in a clear-eyed, purposeful, aggressive person with the erect carriage that goes with mental as well as physical health. Chronic lumbosacral strain commonly occurs in people who treat their bodies like inert shells meant only to house digestive systems and take no special attention. These people usually have a swayback, some degree of humpback and a protruding abdomen as a result of the deterioration of ignored muscles and ligaments. Typically, too, there is poor general hygiene and health habits—constipation, inadequate diet and rest and so on.

Women are most often affected by this condition, and housewives are particularly susceptible. I'm certain high heels and girdles play a role (we discussed heels and posture in Chapter 6). While the wearing of a properly fitted corset or girdle could conceivably be of some benefit in supporting the flabby muscles in these women, many do their housework without wearing their girdles, which they keep for "going out."

THE TREATMENT OF CHRONIC LUMBOSACRAL STRAIN

Once the doctor is certain there is no other condition masquerading as this low back strain and causing the symptoms, he will prescribe postural exercises to increase the strength of the low back and abdominal muscles, as we describe in Chapter 19. Normal weight must be restored and maintained if the sufferer is overweight. Enough rest is important, too, and should include eight hours of sleep a night, along with an hour's bed rest in the afternoon. The mattress should be firm enough to support the body without sagging in the low back region; a plywood board between spring and matress can correct a moderate sag, and there are special orthopedic mattresses available. Firm straight chairs should be used to support the back, and an auto seat back frame if much driving is done. The most important factor is correct posture, but it's also wise to learn to lift things properly and protect the low back, as described in the last chapter.

THE ACUTE LUMBOSACRAL STRAIN

This differs from the chronic form in every way. For one thing, the acute form is caused by an injury to the low back—lifting excessive loads or doing this in the wrong way, some direct trauma to the back or a fall in which the muscles are strained. The acute disorder is also different in its cause, its symptoms, disability and even its treatment.

Whatever sets the particular condition off will produce immediate discomfort. Often, though, the initial pain, which isn't too bad and is felt chiefly as stiffness of the low back, is largely due to muscle spasm. The victim may keep on working or even indulge in exercises in the hope that this will "work out" the condition. While it may often do so, for some reason we don't fully understand, this time it's different. Now it just gets rapidly worse until the pain is so excruciating that the victim is literally paralyzed—he can't move and can barely breathe; he doesn't dare move his toes or even his eyeballs. The pain in these sufferers is so bad that you mustn't touch their beds, for the pain will be agonizing.

However, the average acute lumbosacral strain is not nearly as bad as this and is commonly a low back discomfort; it's usually worse on one side, with the most severe pain often localized to a sharply limited area. Bending forward increases discomfort, and there is limited mobility of the lumbar spine. When the muscles involved are just on one side, bending will be more painful away from the side of the spasm.

THE TREATMENT OF ACUTE LUMBOSACRAL STRAIN

When these patients are wheeled into the hospital totally paralyzed by their pain, the trick is not to nickel and dime them with mild analgesics but to hit them hard with immediate medication (usually narcotics) to get the muscle spasm to relax. Within a few days these sufferers are amazed at how well they feel, and they're invariably more impressed with this than if I'd done the world's most spectacular and amazing surgery. Yet I really haven't done anything for them that requires special skills. In fact, doctors the world over treat acute lumbosacral strain the same way—with rest and medication to ease the discomfort—and these patients do get better.

Acute lumbosacral strain is a muscular condition involving any or all of the muscles below the chest level. These muscles interdigitate so much that if one becomes tight or spastic (goes into spasm), the others will pick it up and do the same. Muscle spasm produces pain, and this pain then produces more spasm. In some way the physician has to break up this cycle, and it doesn't really matter how, whether with rest or medication or heat or cold. When the condition is mild, the sufferer is likely to treat it himself, and Chapter 18 gives you the home remedies I suggest you keep available for the purpose.

Actually this is a self-limiting disease so that almost anything you do that is pain-relieving will make the patient better. But the real trick is to make him better faster and make it easier for him. Heat, cold, massage and even spinal manipulation all have a place, and your doctor can tell which is the one to use for *you*. The most dangerous time in this disease is when the sufferer starts to feel good because these are usually vigorous people who want to get back to work. In fact, they get into these extreme conditions because they didn't want to bother with doctors in the first place and so are impatient with medical care once they're feeling better.

It's best for the victim of acute low back strain to stay in bed a couple of extra days because if he gets out too early, there's a good chance of recurrence. Sometimes, too, a light canvas support for the low back is wise so the victim can then resume his job and still minimize the likelihood of a recurrence. Exercises are also valuable, starting with some gentle muscle-stretching ones. The doctor should supervise these exercises because too much too soon may well set off the whole cycle again. This danger of too much too soon must be kept in mind because it's also true of the return to any form of activities—whether housework, household repairs, work at the job, sports or anything else.

But there is also a danger here of excessive rest, for this may not only prolong the recovery period but even create a so-called low back neurosis in which the person comes to regard himself as an invalid. This may eventually even progress to a permanent disability, and the wise doctor is careful to tread a fine line between too much too soon and the danger of excessive rest or confinement.

Chapter 9

THE NEW WORLD OF THE SLIPPED DISK:
Fact vs. Fiction, Surgery or No Surgery

To MOST people the very term "spinal disk" means only one thing—big trouble. It conjures up a picture of the slipped disk: some sort of severe accident or injury to the back; almost irreparable damage done; immediate major back surgery required, with a lifetime of suffering invalidism to follow it all. Finally, most people regard the slipped disk as a rarity, something that only happens to someone else, to an unfortunate few. All of which adds up to a very bleak and gloomy picture.

This is the common picture—only it's far more fiction than fact. Certainly there are elements of truth in this picture, but overall it's wrong. Disk disease (a much better term since disks never do "slip") affects nearly every one of us (if we live to be over sixty), and more than a quarter of a million Americans were in the hospital for this condition in 1970. Today we *don't* operate as readily for slipped disks as we once did; surgery is much less common now than it has been and there's also a new injection which may well make much of even this limited surgery obsolete before too long. So this chapter will discount much of the popular mythology about slipped disks or herniated disks or disk disease—and spell out the reality instead.

How Long Have Slipped Disks Been Around?

Probably since man began walking on two legs—but we

have actual written evidence of the presence of the disk disease going back some 5,000 years. For the Edwin Smith Papyrus discussed earlier describes a technique very much like one many doctors still use (medically known as Lasegue's sign) for diagnosing sciatica and disk disease. Intervertebral disks have been known for nearly half a century, while a treatise on sciatica appeared more than 200 years ago.

In 1883 Sir William Macewen, professor of surgery at the University of Glasgow, performed the first laminectomy, the operation used for disk surgery. In this procedure the rear portion of the spine was removed to expose the spinal canal. First done for a boy whose curvature of the spine was producing problems, the result was excellent, for Sir William relieved the pressure on the spinal cord. It took a brilliant innovative surgeon to dare this surgery initially, but Macewen was also one of the first to drain a brain abscess. When surgeons were losing virtually 100 percent of their patients with this operation, Macewen got twenty-three recoveries in twenty-four of his early patients with this abscess, surgery for which is still dangerous despite antibiotics.

Early in this century, surgeons used Macewen's laminectomy to remove fibrous masses which were pressing on the spinal nerves as they came off the cord (as we described in Chapter 2). However, what they were removing was a matter of speculation. Some thought the masses were tumors, while others believed they were developmental growths. No one was completely sure until August, 1934, when a report appeared in the prestigious *New England Journal of Medicine* by Dr. Jason Mixter and Dr. Joseph S. Barr, Sr., an orthopedic surgeon, both of Massachusetts General Hospital. These doctors told of a series of successful operations to remove the disk material which had ruptured into the spinal canal and thus to relieve the patients' low back pain and sciatica.

Actually this was not the first such operation, and Mixter and Barr were neither the original disk surgeons nor the first to remove herniated lumbar disks. They were the first, however, to recognize this was a herniated disk they had removed, a condition in which mechanical stress caused the disk material to protrude and produce nerve root pressure. In short, they clarified the disease, making it a distinct entity with a specific clinical picture, clear-cut signs and symptoms, and provided a good description of their surgery. By doing all this, they popularized the condition in the minds of physicians, and the "era of the disk" had begun.

Other articles quickly followed Mixter and Barr's, and the medical profession became increasingly involved with this new concept, disk disease. In fact, physicians were affected by what the young training fighter pilots of World War II suffered—target fixation: In their first few dogfights these fledglings so riveted their attention on the enemy that even after he was destroyed, the young pilots couldn't free themselves of this concentration, often ending in a midair collison or following so closely on their enemy's tail that they crashed to the ground with him.

Only with experience did these pilots learn to maintain a sense of objectivity in combat and avoid target fixation. After Mixter and Barr, the medical profession developed the same target fixation and became so enmeshed in this new concept of the ruptured disk that physicians lost all awareness of the other possible causes for low back pain and looked only for herniated disks.

It's really just recently that the profession has begun to escape this entrapment and regain its objectivity in assessing low back problems. The same target fixation led to the excessive disk surgery in the early days of this era, but the pendulum is now swinging back, and physicians are finally reaching a more neutral ground, one not so biased toward lumbar disk surgery as the single or chief answer to the low back disorders that patients suffer.

The Slipped Disk: What It Is and How It Happens

The spinal disk serves two functions: to provide mobility to the spine and to act as a shock absorber. If you will recall our earlier discussions, the center, or nucleus pulposus, is a loose network of fibrous tissue within a semitransparent muco-protein gel with a gelatinous consistency, 90 percent of which is water. With age this water content drops to about 70 per-cent, and the degenerated nucleus turns denser, more fibrous and opaque. The annulus fibrosus is a dense fibrocar-tilage outer envelope of some dozen concentric rings with the fibers of one layer running at an angle to those of the preceding layer. The disk also has top and bottom layers of cartilage to hold it together.

The annulus is thinner and less firm along its back part,

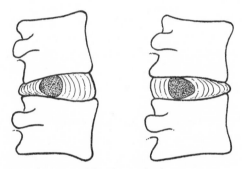

Figure 7. Normal lumbar spinal movement pro-duces a slight protrusion of the annulus fibrosus.

where it's closest to to the spinal canal with its vital nerves. When you bend over, the nucleus acts almost like a ball bear-ing, permitting the vertebra above and below to rock on the nucleus. When up-and-down pressures occur (in lifting heavy weights, for example), the nucleus flattens, and there is a compensatory stretching of the annular fibers. The disk may even protrude slightly with stress, but it is held in place by the ligaments (a stronger one in front, a weaker one be-hind, so any extrusion goes toward the rear, where the spinal canal lies).

But this is no weak sister. In a young adult the normal in-tervertebral disk will yield and deform only at pressures over 1,400 pounds, but in an older individual this occurs with only

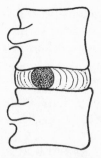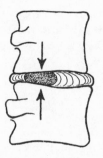

Figure 8. Axial vertebral compression produces slight flattening of the nucleus and a compensatory "stretching" of the annular fibers.

about 350 pounds. It has been found that the protruded disk (the herniated or slipped disk) of a young man shows a loss of water, increased density and a more fibrous nature; this is what one would expect in the normal disk of the older person. Some believe that disk degeneration actually represents a premature aging process.

Tests have shown that the normal disk is actually more resistant to trauma than bone and is not what gives under extreme pressure, or the vertebrae will fracture before the disk. Clinical experience confirms this, for compression fractures of the lumbar spine are often seen in certain accidents. Take snowmobile injuries occurring when the buttocks are raised from the seat and then smashed down when shooting over an embankment, or a fall on ice where the feet go out from under the person, who then lands on the buttocks, or the seat ejection of jet pilots by catapults. In these accidents the vertebrae fracture, not the disks.

All of which makes the change in even young protruded disks significant, for this may indicate that the slipped or herniated disk is really a degenerated or prematurely old disk. And this would make sense simply because some people spend their whole lives doing the heaviest work—stevedores or movers, for example—and never have a ruptured disk.

Yet a desk worker may get one by bending over to pick up a paperweight or leaning forward to brush his teeth.

What actually happens is that some mechanical stress causes the nucleus to squeeze through the weakened annulus. Since the back part of the annulus is thinner and weaker, the nucleus will break through—rupture, herniate, extrude, "slip"—at the back. But here the spinal ligaments, too, are weaker than those in front and lie in the spinal canal. If the extruded portion of the nucleus is toward the back corner, it will squeeze the nerve root that comes off the spinal cord (one of the thirty-one paired spinal nerves) and press it against the protecting bone. The effect will show up in the skin area that the nerve supplies. Thus, when the sciatic nerve is squeezed, you will get an effect—pain or numbness or pins and needles and the like—in the buttocks, the low back, down the back of the leg and even into the foot—in short, typical sciatica.

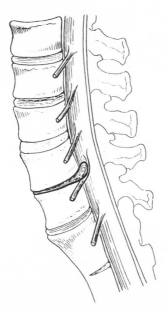

Figure 9. Herniated L4-5 disk causing nerve root compression.

However, should there be a massive pushing out (extrusion) of the nucleus, squeezing through all along the back of the annulus and compressing the spinal cord or the cauda equina (the group of spinal nerves coming off the end of the spinal cord and running down through the lumbar and sacral spinal column), then the effect is a major emergency.

A forty-year-old man complained of some moderate low back pain and sciatica for years, had been treated conservatively and was responding well (we'll go into treatment later in the chapter) until he leaned over the sink to brush his teeth one day. At that instant he experienced a sudden excruciating low back pain, weakness in both legs and an inability to urinate. Special X rays confirmed the diagnosis of a massive disk extrusion; immediate surgery relieved the pressure before permanent nerve damage was done. Wait in this situation, and the neurological symptoms (the paralysis of the leg and sphincter muscles which control urination and defecation) are more likely to persist.

How Common Is the Degenerated and the Herniated Disk?

A recent study of the spinal disks of sixty-three subjects from fourteen to eighty years of age with relatively "normal" backs and without symptoms was revealing—and startling. Those from fourteen to thirty-four years of age had ninety percent of their disks normal and ten percent degenerated (even at this young age). In those from thirty-five to fifty-nine years of age only 25 percent had *normal* disks. And of those over sixty years of age only five percent had normal disks. It's significant that most patients with herniated disks are between thirty and fifty, which would seem to indicate again that something more than age or injury is involved, that some intrinsic disk weakness must be present.

In a national study it was found that an estimated 277,000 patients were hospitalized in 1970 with ruptured intervertebral disks. Incidentally, some 85 percent of these were low back (lumbar), which fits in well with the estimate that nine out of ten spinal problems are actually low back. This same study revealed that 128,000 operations were performed for ruptured disks in 1970. Clearly the herniated disk is a major problem, and the National Center for Health Statistics reports that nearly 2,000,000 Americans in 1969 suffered with slipped or ruptured disks.

How Your Doctor Diagnoses Disk Disease: The Examination

In most instances of herniated disks your doctor will quickly recognize the condition from a combination of what has happened to you, what you feel and what his simple examination shows. He will use that little rubber hammer you're undoubtedly familiar with from having your knees tapped by doctors over the years, a couple of pins and perhaps a little rotating wheel with sharp points sticking out and, finally, an ordinary tape measure. He will use just these simple painless things, your history and his eyes (seeing how you move, for example, when he asks you to walk toward him on your heels and then away from him on your toes) to diagnose the condition.

He will have you bending and twisting, check the strength and working of the muscles of your legs and even your toes, tap your knees and the back of your heels with his little rubber hammer (which is why the neurologists, the nerve specialists, came to be called, in the medical profession, the rubber hammer boys) to check your reflexes. Your doctor will also measure the length of your legs and the thickness of each thigh or calf to compare with the other to see if there's been any atrophy from nerve damage; then check your sensations with a wisp of cotton and gently test areas he suspects, using the sharp end of a pin and the wheel we mentioned. He'll move your legs in various ways, one of which may be a leg-raising test devised by Dr. Ernest Charles Lasegue in 1964 for sciatica—and mentioned 5,000 years ago in the Edwin Smith Papyrus.

Only if there is a question of what the problem really is or if surgery is being considered seriously will special X rays be taken. These are the myelograms which have gained an unnecessarily evil reputation since they are actually both safe and painless in the vast majority of instances today (they are discussed in detail in Chapter 13) and the diskograms to show the disks themselves or in connection with the use of papaya juice discussed later in this chapter. An ordinary X ray too may likely be taken, but this is no cause for concern. However, it's impossible to diagnose a slipped disk with this, although it does have other uses.

The Symptoms of the Herniated or Slipped Disk

The commonest and the most typical symptom in the patient who develops a herniated disk is severe low back and leg pain. This pain may develop for no known cause or reason, or it may be related to some trauma, such as lifting something very heavy or twisting or falling. The pain may run across the buttock and down the leg, even into the foot. This is sciatica and is due to an irritation of the sciatic nerve or pressure on it. About three-quarters of patients with sciatica also have paresthesia (strange skin sensations such as tingling, itching, burning, feelings of pins and needles or hot or cold), numbness, paralysis or just weakness. There may also be a loss of control over bladder or bowel or both. All this may occur when the nucleus herniates or ruptures through the fibers of the annulus and then presses against either nerve roots or the entire nerve contents of the spinal canal. The result also depends in part on your good fortune. If you have a narrow spinal canal, it won't take very much extruded nuclear material to produce disastrous effects, whereas if yours is a large roomy canal, a limited herniation will produce very little effect.

The whole process likely begins (and we're far from certain even now just how this whole thing happens or why) with an alteration of the mucoprotein content of the nucleus, along with a softening and microscopic swelling of the annular fibers. With the nucleus degenerated and more fibrous and with reduced elasticity of both this and the annulus, the disk is less prepared to take stress or pressure without bulging. The actual rupture of the annulus may be a gradual process as a result of slow disintegration or happen suddenly from a specific trauma or stress.

With these changes go a predisposition and weakness so that it may take only a sudden lumbar bend or flexion (say, to tie one's shoes or to lean forward in shaving) to cause the nucleus to break through the annulus and discharge degenerated fragments into the spinal canal or to one side of the central posterior ligament to press on the spinal nerve root. Actually about nine out of ten herniated lumbar disks occur at the lowest two interspaces of the spine, between the fourth and fifth lumbar vertebrae, and between the fifth lumbar vertebra and the sacrum, probably because this is the area of greatest mechanical stress. A double herniation, or the simultaneous rupture of both these lower disks, occurs in about one in ten slipped disk victims. Incidentally, now you see that a "slipped disk" never really slips, but the term is so well known to both public and profession alike that we all still use it for convenience.

Most clear-cut cases of herniated disks can be readily diagnosed on a combination of symptoms and physical examination. But I have found something else in a study of my own. I went through records of patients on whom I had to operate for herniated disks between 1961 and 1970 and pulled out 1,000 consecutive and unselected cases for study. These presented an interesting picture of the herniated disk victim: the sufferers ranged in age from fourteen to seventy-nine with an average age of forty-two, and they were 769 men and 231 women (three times as many men as expected).

Of these 1,000 patients, 643 recalled backaches before their herniated disks occurred. But we don't know what produces these early symptoms. They may be early changes in the nucleus that increases the stress on the annulus outer fibers which contain pain nerves. Typically the pain was intermittent and included 192 with "severe" pain, which would vary from "hardly noticeable" to "extremely severe"; 320 with "moderate" pain, which usually occurred on strenuous activities but occasionally was spontaneous; and 131 with "mild" pain, such as a "mild ache," a "tired feeling in my back."

It might be useful to note that the moderate pain was precipitated by such exertion as an unusual weekend of sports, gardening or prolonged stooping, spring housecleaning or heavy lifting and usually improved with rest or a few aspirins.

Characteristically, the herniated disk patient will have these symptoms before the disk ruptures. But sometimes the preexisting symptoms can be as little as "I always had a weak back," "I was a bit stiff on arising in the morning" or stiffness after a long car trip. The pain is often so insidious in onset that many patients are unable to recall when it started. The symptoms were present anywhere from eight weeks to five years before herniation. And while four of these 131 patients with mild preexisting backaches had been hospitalized before for low back pain, in three of them the hospitalization was the only severe backache they had ever had. The sufferers most often tie these symptoms and difficulties in with some trauma in the past. Of the 1,000 patients, 764 could recall an injury, but this varied widely from a fall from a ladder over ten feet high to bending forward over a sink to wash one's face. And sciatica was present either with or without back pain in 964 of these patients.

The symptoms of the herniated disk itself are a wholly different ball game. This may be a pain virtually as bad as that of a lumbosacral strain with the patient unable to move and in agonizing pain when touched or moved, however gently. Such severe pain is happily rare, and most patients are in great discomfort but can tolerate their pain for a time, particularly with medical help. The pain may be in the low back, and usually is, but it may also involve the buttocks or legs or feet, usually on one side since only when there is a double extrusion, one on each side of the posterior ligament, or a massive one right across the middle are both sides affected. But there may also be neurological symptoms: These may be complete or partial paralysis of one or both legs and feet, weakness of leg and foot muscles with difficulty in walking; the bladder or bowel or both may be incontinent; reflexes such as knee jerk or ankle jerk may be reduced or absent.

For example, a woman in her mid-thirties had had no significant low back dysfunction until a fall was followed by severe intractable low back and right sciatic pain. The ankle jerk was absent, and the side of her right foot was numb. A myelogram revealed three disk protrusions—at the disk spaces of L3–4, L4–5 and L5–S1. The symptoms were due to the lowest herniated disk, so I removed only this one, and the sufferer recovered well. Because this woman will probably be predisposed to low back problems in the future, I advised her to change her job to a less physically demanding one than the one she had. But I don't believe in "prophylactic" disk removal, and patients are best served by not removing the herniated disks which cause no symptoms.

The New Approach to Herniated Disks: Surgery or No Surgery?

With the advent of the era of the disk in 1934, when Mixter and Barr's article appeared, the medical profession became deeply involved in disk surgery. The surgery itself is not a particularly formidable procedure when it's performed by a competent, experienced surgeon (we'll discuss how to find one in Chapter 12). Many surgeons employ spinal anesthesia for the operation, but I prefer intravenous sodium pentothal ("truth serum," given by injection into a vein and often used by dentists today) along with nitrous oxide by inhalation ("laughing gas," long the favorite of dentistry for its simplicity and safety), and this is probably the majority choice in lumbar disk surgery.

The operation is often referred to by patients and doctors

alike as laminectomy, but this is a misnomer since it means literally the complete removal of a lamina, which is usually avoided by most experienced surgeons today. The aim is to avoid weakening the spine by preserving as much bone as possible and keeping the spine as intact and "natural" as possible. The lamina is the back part of the vertebra protecting the spinal canal, and the new approach is to slip the surgical instruments in between the lamina and remove the herniated disk and all other degenerated disk fragments. To do this more conservative procedure, the surgeon has to work in a space not much larger than a keyhole, which is difficult but worthwhile since it will be more beneficial for the patient.

Sometimes slivers of bone from a bone bank or the patient's own hip are placed behind and alongside the involved vertebrae to gain a spinal fusion, or permanent fusing of the vertebrae on each side. This, however, limits the amount of back mobility, and indications for spinal fusion are distinctly limited; the surgery itself and its later effects can cause sufficient problems to make this operation reserved to those instances where it *must* be used.

The success rate of simple disk excision (disk surgery) is high, and where the criteria for surgery are proper (certain symptoms and adequate X ray and myelographic studies), there is less than a 10 percent failure rate. The patient who undergoes disk surgery is up and walking around the day after his surgery and released from the hospital a week after the operation. However, there is a minimum of six weeks' convalescence before the desk worker can return to his job, and twelve weeks for the manual laborer. The patient is frequently fitted with a spinal brace or corset which he wears whenever out of bed for twelve weeks.

Too much disk surgery is being done in the United States (surgeons are much more conservative abroad), and there are a variety of reasons for this, but since this is a complicated subject, I prefer to leave it to Chapter 12. There, too, you will find this whole question of every kind of surgery explored, along with how you can protect yourself against unnecessary surgery, how you can go about finding the proper surgeon and the like.

If you should have a herniated disk, it does *not* mean that you must undergo surgery. The most recent change in our thinking is away from surgery because it is finally striking home to everybody that disk surgery is not the answer for a very large number of patients with back trouble. In fact, there are many patients who have been subjected to surgery and have not done very well. The medical profession is beginning to realize that disk surgery is not the panacea it was once thought to be.

We're now taking a step or two backward and being much more patient, trying to get a little further with conservative management of these sufferers and holding off taking our patients to the operating room. Many do eventually get better, do quite well and don't require surgery after all.

The Conservative Nonsurgical Treatment

If you can cope with the pain, you don't need surgery. Operations are only to allow people to lead meaningful and full lives, so they don't just stay in bed all the time, so they can get into the car and visit Mother or go fishing, so they can go shopping and stand in the check-out line without having to sit down for a while and start all over again at the end. That's the *only* reason for surgery for ordinary disk disease. When there are the neurological symptoms—say, the slight foot weakness or the reduced knee jerk or the slight numbness—and surgery removes the pressure on the nerve, the symptoms will often still remain afterward.

Virtually every patient with acute symptoms of lumbar disk disease is helped by bed rest and made worse by activity. So long as you're in the upright position you're putting weight on that little piece of gristle, that disk, and there is no way for its little bulge to recede. But the sufferer often finds himself stiff and uncomfortable after a period of inactivity while light activity makes him feel "limber." Goaded by this, the patient may intentionally increase his activity—and end up with a flare-up that is completely incapacitating.

An electrical hospital bed at home or in the hospital can give a slight head elevation, which is better for the back and for the morale since you can watch TV or visitors. A side position is allowed, with hips and knees bent. But bed rest is strictly enforced except for a daily trip or two to the bathroom. Gradually the bed rest is reduced as the symptoms disappear until the patient is entirely up except for sleep.

Traction is a time-honored procedure that is used today. This consists of a canvas girdle which hugs the hips and pelvis and is attached to weights of fifteen pounds dangling over the foot of the bed. Physicians are divided over the use of traction for lumbar disk disease. The majority believe that properly applied pelvic traction will straighten out the lumbar curve (the low back hollow, or lumbar lordosis); this will, in turn, change the vertebral alignment so that the herniated disk can slip back into its original position and thus take the pressure off the affected nerve root.

However, there are some physicians who are either uncertain or frankly skeptical about the benefits of traction, believing that any improvement is actually due to the bed rest involved. But even some of these skeptics will still use traction—as an excuse to keep the patient in bed and to give him the feeling that at least "something is being done for me."

Both heat and ice are also used, depending on the results and the sufferer, for ice will work on one patient, while another patient will be helped only by heat. Massage and manipulation, too, are ancient forms of therapy but debatable, and again help may come from either or neither of them. The way all these are used in a variety of low back disorders will be detailed in Chapters 17 and 18.

Low back exercises and correct posture have an important role once the acute stage of lumbar disk disease has subsided.

Essential in the conservative management of this problem are the many things you must learn—if you suffer with this condition—in order to make life easier for yourself, it is hoped, and to prevent problems. But these things apply to many areas of low back dysfunction and are best covered in the overall discussion in Chapters 19 and 20.

The doctor will go over with you—after an acute attack of disk disease—the activities of your daily life (whether you can indulge in contact sports or heavy gardening, what exercises are best for *you,* even whether you should change your job and so on). Much will depend on whether your job is physical and how long you will have it (you may be ready for a promotion to a supervisory position and merely need to get by for a year or two), or your task may be housework, and this too must be planned with your doctor if you are to avoid another painful spell.

In the majority of patients with disk disease today we *can* avoid surgery—if they are willing to cooperate. There is even a new treatment with exciting promise. In the last few years an injection of the juice of the papaya fruit (chymopapain) into herniated disks has shown remarkable results. It has made thousands of cases of surgery unnecessary, for it has relieved the disk condition. But it is a complicated matter that you should know a good deal about, so I've devoted Chapter 16 to it, for it may well be a major breakthrough in this field.

What I Think of Disk Surgery

There is nothing more drastic, more positive, more final than surgery, and there is no substitute for a normal back that has never had surgery. Once you make an incision and put a scar there, once you take away even a little bone and remove a portion of a disk, the back never comes back to normal. Sometimes surgery is the best alternative—but only when alternatives have been tried and have failed. When

there is no other choice and the indications are clear and un-
mistakable, then surgery can be highly successful, and there
need be no trouble in the future using it.

My Business Is Giving You Six Slices, Not the Whole Loaf

Everybody wants the whole loaf. All patients want to be
able to do all they ever did before they had disk disease, to
run and play and work without limitations. But I'm in the
business of giving you only six slices instead of the whole
loaf. Once you've had disk disease, you have to accept limitations to avoid surgery, and if you have surgery, you'll still
have some limitations in the degree of your activities, all depending on your circumstances.

Chapter 10

ARTHRITIS, INFECTIONS AND TUMORS OF THE LOW BACK SPINE

THIS IS a story of Betty Ford and of gold, of drug addicts and a dream of all mankind. It's a story of medical miracles, of magic chemicals that work and of others that don't. It's a story of a 200,000,000-year-old disease that we still don't understand, although almost all of us will suffer with it if we live even to anywhere near retirement age, and of a particularly despicable element in our society that feeds on sufferers to the tune of a half billion dollars a year.

True, the outlook for these diseases of the spine varies widely, and so does the treatment. But one thing is the same: All can cause suffering and disability; all can worry and distress the victims. But here are their stories, along with some sources of available help or information.

Arthritis of the Spine

The figures on this disorder are truly overwhelming: At least 50,000,000 Americans are estimated to have some arthritis and 17,000,000 of these suffer enough with it to need medical attention. Each year it claims another 250,000 new victims, and the cost to the nation runs annually to nearly $4 billion. And 97 percent of those past the age of sixty have enough arthritis to show on X rays.

However, arthritis is nothing new—the dinosaur of 200 million years ago suffered with osteoarthritis (spondylitis deformans) of his spine, and early Paleolithic man or preman

117

of some 2,500,000 years ago suffered with rheumatoid arthritis. Whether it was Piltdown or Neanderthal or Heidelberg man, all show evidence that arthritis plagued men then as now. What was once called cave gout (arthritis deformans or rheumatoid arthritis) can be found in Egyptian mummies or the remains of ancient Incas, in the early North American Indians or the Pleistocene cave bears. Not long ago, First Lady Betty Ford had to cancel a trip to accompany the President to a Martinique conference with French President Valery Giscard d'Estaing because her low back osteoarthritis flared up, as it has in the past. Mrs. Ford had to remain home for hot packs and massages.

WHAT IS ARTHRITIS?

The word comes from the Greek *arthron,* meaning joint, and the medical suffix *itis,* meaning inflammation. So arthritis is literally the inflammation of a joint. However, the term actually covers close to a hundred conditions causing pain in the joints or connective tissues of the body, and not all are actually inflammatory.

Arthritis has frequently been called everybody's disease, and as we've seen, this is true, sooner or later, although women make up two-thirds of the "arthritic" population. What most disturbs sufferers about arthritis is their fear of becoming crippled. In the low back, there are essentially only three forms of arthritis which strike this area to any degree: osteoarthritis, ankylosing spondylitis and rheumatoid arthritis.

OSTEOARTHRITIS OF THE SPINE

The specialists in arthritic problems (the rheumatologists) prefer to call this condition degenerative joint disease, and this explains what it is. It is a degenerative condition, and the most popular explanation is that it's a disease of "wear and tear." But this doesn't hold up too well, for you find it in the fingers, and they don't carry any weight. Still, we have nothing better to substitute for this explanation, although metabolic causes are being studied.

Osteoarthritis does affect the low back since this area of the body carries weight, as we have seen. But again there is some confusion here, for the spines that show the most X ray changes often have far less pain than severe sufferers who often show only very minor radiographic changes. In the low back the complaints are twofold: pain and a loss of mobility. The sufferer may have difficulty in bending and a stiff spine to a widely varying and very individual degree. The pain may be just low back, or it may occasionally radiate to the thigh and sometimes have a sciatic type of distribution. But worse than the pain and the limitation of motion is the terror that this will make the sufferer a total cripple—a fear that is almost never realized.

The treatment is relatively simple—low back exercises to protect the spine and to keep it supple—but these, as well as the daily activities, are best individually prescribed. Correct posture is important, and a hard bed is best for sleeping; activities and weight bearing may be limited, and supports or braces or corsets prescribed. Aspirin is still the chief medication, and it reduces the inflammation in the joints at the same time that it relieves the pain. There are other new antiinflammatory drugs, but aspirin is still the mainstay of arthritis fighting. Heat, too, may help, and when the condition really gets bad, the sufferer just has to get off his feet for a couple of days or a week. Sometimes traction is used.

But more than anything else is the reassurance that only the doctor can give—that the sufferer will not be crippled but may well be hampered and often limited. It's something that has to be lived with until the day we understand more about this disease.

ANKYLOSING SPONDYLITIS: THE BAMBOO SPINE

This is a male chauvinist disease! It favors men over women, 10 to 1, and it runs in families; at the 1973 Arthritis

Foundation meeting four Northeastern doctors reported on a single family in which there were eight diagnosed cases of this disorder in three generations. It's also a tragic disease in that it strikes at the height of youth, in the teens and the twenties and only rarely after thirty. It sneaks up on its victims and can cripple the young adult virtually without warning. Ankylosing spondylitis comes from the Greek *ankylosis,* or stiffening of a joint, plus *spondylos,* or vertebra, and *itis,* meaning inflammation.

This brings us back to our old friend the intervertebral disk. For ankylosing spondylitis (AS) causes a bonelike hardening of the annulus fibrosus along with changes in the intervertebral joints similar to those of rheumatoid arthritis, of which AS may be a form. It starts off with low back discomfort, episodes of stiffness or aching more often apparent after staying in one position for some time and particularly on awakening in the morning. AS is so vague that its victims usually don't seek medical help at first and later don't recall just when it all began.

As time passes, however, the periods of discomfort become more severe, and the victim may even be awakened from a sound sleep during the night by the pain. Unlike most back problems, it isn't particularly aggravated by activity. About three-quarters of these sufferers have some form of sciatica, usually during the early phases of the disease. The increasingly severe episodes of pain over the years will coincide with the growing rigidity of the spine until the entire vertebral column becomes rigid and fixed and there appears a limited ability to expand the chest.

There is no known treatment today which can stop the progression of this disorder, which starts with the sacroiliac joints and works its way up through the lumbar vertebrae all the way to the head. AS usually takes ten to twenty years for the classical poker-back type of deformity, the hunchback, to develop. However, the disease may on occasion remain limited to the sacroiliac joints, or on the contrary, it may move rapidly upward.

The outlook for the control of pain and the maintenance

of ability to work and function is usually good, and three-quarters or more of these patients are able to find full employment. Aspirin is still important in the treatment of this disease, but phenylbutazone and indomethacin—anti-inflammatory drugs—are now also being used. Special postural exercises are individually prescribed and very beneficial, and heat is helpful.

RHEUMATOID ARTHRITIS

This is just the opposite of AS in that it strikes women three times as often as men. Moreover, it's the most serious, the most painful and the most damaging and crippling of the arthritides. One of the most striking features of this dread disease is its extreme individuality, for it varies greatly from patient to patient. It shows a startling tendency to undergo spontaneous remissions (seemingly disappearing completely) and severe flare-ups. Many times the original condition is mild and disappears completely or is confined to just a few joints with little or no permanent damage done.

In general, though, the pain is often excruciating, and joints swell and stiffen until they can no longer be used. There may be generalized symptoms such as fatigue, and rheumatoid arthritis can attack the heart and lungs, skin and spleen, as well as other organs and tissues. Joints throughout the body may be attacked, and in the spine the facet joints may be assaulted with the same destruction and damage and pain as elsewhere. Of particular danger is the destruction of the joint between the atlas and the axis, leading to a partial dislocation and even spinal cord compression (pressure) with very serious effects. This arthritis can cause severe low back pain when the disks degenerate from it, and there can be severe effects on the spines of children in particular.

The cause is still a mystery, as is the erratic behavior it follows. Treatment is individual and requires an all-out attack, but its efficacy is still markedly limited. Aspirin is the most widely used drug here, as with the other arthritides. During the 1920s a French rheumatologist, Dr. Jacques Forestier, thought that arthritis resembled tuberculosis, for which gold was then being prescribed, and so tried that precious metal in injections for rheumatoid arthritis. It was gradually shown that the two diseases are very different, and gold is ineffective in tuberculosis, but the metal has worked for rheumatoid arthritis. Weekly gold injections for ten to twelve weeks may produce gradual lessening of the pain, stiffness, fatigue and other symptoms of rheumatoid arthritis—when it works and if it doesn't have unfortunate side effects.

So both gold and aspirin, along with many other drugs, exercises, rest, heat and surgery, are used in this terrible disease. But we still have a long way to go to conquer this ravaging disorder. But some of the most tragic aspects of the arthritides lie not in the disease.

THE QUACKERY OF ARTHRITIS—AND SOME REAL HELP

If you suffer from arthritis, the chances are that you have fallen for some kind of "cure" or "miraculous remedy" or whatever at some time or other. Almost every arthritic has.

This is the lowest and most despicable kind of fraud there is, for it robs arthritis victims of almost $500,000,000 every year and, even worse, steals precious time during which the disease may be getting worse and during which the condition might be getting help.

Before you get involved in arthritis diets (there are none except for gout), "guaranteed" magic devices or whatnot, check with your doctor or the Arthritis Foundation either locally or at its national headquarters, 1212 Avenue of the Americas, New York, N.Y. 10036. In fact, if you suffer with this disease, information is available at the Foundation or the National Institute of Arthritis, Metabolism and Infectious Disease (in Bethesda, Maryland 20014).

Infections of the Spine

This is a problem which often escapes the physician's notice simply because infections of the lumbar spine are not common. Yet they do occur often enough to warrant consideration when the doctor makes a diagnosis. The infection itself may be acute and pus-producing—owing to bacteria—or be chronic, owing to tuberculosis or to a fungus (mycotic). Spinal infections occur more commonly in adults than in children and as often in men as in women. These infections can be blood-borne (bacteria brought by the bloodstream) from some distant source such as a respiratory or genitourinary (bladder or kidney or prostate) infection, or they can idiopathic (of unknown origin or self-originated) or may even occur after spinal surgery.

In general, spinal infections—apart from those that follow spinal surgery—usually do not involve the nerve roots, and in many instances the symptoms are confined to the low back. The nontuberculous ("tubercular" actually means nodular, not the disease) infections have a number of special characteristics in children, demanding a different approach from that in adults. The intervertebral disk infections in children commonly attack the lower thoracic and the lumbar disks and generally run a milder course than in adults, in whom any place in the spine may be involved.

In adults, spinal infections follow a more insidious and a more destructive course. Pyogenic spondylitis (technically a pus-producing inflammation of one or more vertebrae) may appear spontaneously with no recognizable infection elsewhere. We believe that the germs spread from a center within the vertebral body, but the exact cause of the infection is still in doubt.

Staphylococcus (staph) is one of the causes of this infection and produces the widespread spinal bone destruction commonly seen after hip joint surgery. In these infections there is severe pain in the low back, aggravated by any movement or exertion and not relieved by rest. The cause of the pain is unknown, and X ray changes don't show up until a month or so after the pain begins. In some patients the spine becomes fused, while in others meningitis may develop.

Only rarely is a disk space (the space between two vertebrae and occupied by the disk) abscess seen. One I recall was a sixty-year-old woman who suffered excruciating low back pain with sciatica, which was aggravated by any movements. Surgery was performed, and pus was found in the L5–S1 disk space and proved to be a staph infection. Drained and treated with antibiotics, the condition cleared up without problems, and she returned to work in three months.

These pus-producing infections are much more common in children, and we have already described one in Chapter 7. Actually many children have probably had these infections which were never diagnosed, for they start with simple back pain and lumbar muscle spasm. By the time the X rays show narrowing of the disk space the symptoms are greatly reduced, and the physician will likely be content to let well enough alone and not pursue the diagnosis. However, any abrupt appearance of malaise, fever and low back pain in a child should be a warning of the possibility of intervertebral disk infection.

Some of these arise from known sources such as a skin infection or an appendectomy, but most of the time there is no known source. Staph is the usual germ, and in children under five years of age the first symptoms will be a refusal to walk, along with back pain, irritability, fever and often a loss of appetite and weight loss. There may be tenderness over a small area of the spine, and the child may walk—if he can at all—in a gingerly fashion or may limp. With treatment (antibiotics and bed rest) the disease lasts from two to six weeks and there is a reduced disk space at first. In the younger child this returns to normal in six to twelve weeks, but in the older child there may even be a spontaneous fusion of the vertebrae.

The tuberculous spinal infection is usually the result of the initial lung infection, although medical laboratory workers have been known to contract the disease by scratching or pricking themselves with infected instruments. The tuberculous lumbar spine infection is more gradual in its pattern. There is first a dull, aching low back pain that is made worse by exertion but not helped by rest. There's low back tenderness and an evening rise in temperature, and there are some X ray changes. The vertebrae may become osteoporotic and even collapse. Abscesses may form, and the patient may suffer weakness, weight loss and lack of appetite, even night sweats.

Treatment of the spinal condition involves immobilization with a body spica (a plaster of paris cast encasing the entire trunk) for three months and antituberculous drugs for almost twice that long. Surgery is rarely necessary but would consist of removing the diseased tissues and placing drains for direct instillation of the antituberculous drugs.

Our current epidemic of drug addiction has increased the spinal infection problem to the point where Dr. Michael J. Patzakis of the Los Angeles County–USC Medical Center recently reported diagnosing one such case every month, compared to two or three cases of spinal infections a year. Along with this has come the danger of venereal disease infections, for these conditions, too, have reached epidemic proportions. The drug user is notorious in his use of dirty needles under filthy circumstances for the injection of the drugs he needs so desperately, and this introduces infection into both the body and the bloodstream, producing the spinal infections when the bacteria happen to lodge there.

Another reason for our increase in spinal infections has been the increased crowding in many of large cities with a resultant rise in tuberculosis. And strange things do happen. Only recently the New York *Times* reported that a newborn infant was found to have tuberculosis. A search revealed one of the nurses' aides who cared for newborn infants as the possible source. Tests were advised for 1,200 babies who had come under her care in a six-month period, and two infants were found infected.

Tumors of the Spine

Basically there are two types of tumors: benign and malignant. Benign tumors are those growths that do not invade or destroy the tissues about them, nor do they spread to distant parts of the body (metastasize). Malignant tumors—cancers—are the ones that spread and destroy other tissues both locally and at distant points in the body; moreover, they have a tendency to recur even when they're removed. The exact reason why certain cancers tend to spread to particular places often isn't understood; sometimes it's simply that the blood or lymph vessels are so arranged that it's easy to carry tumor cells to particular places. Both primary (original) and metastatic (spread from elsewhere) tumors involve the bony spines, but the ligaments and disks are rarely affected.

THE BENIGN TUMORS

The hemangioma (from the Greek *haima,* or blood, *angeion,* or vessel, and *onkoma,* or swelling) is a benign tumor made up of newly formed blood vessels and is found in 10 percent of all spines when they are put through careful and thorough anatomical examinations. These tumors occur most often in the lumbar vertebrae and in women almost twice as often as in men. They appear more often with age, and most are found unexpectedly during autopsies with no symptoms at all during life.

However, the hemangiomas do hollow out the vertebrae, and large tumors may even cause a ballooning of the sides of the vertebrae, but fractures are rare. Only occasionally are there any symptoms, and these usually occur only because the vertebral body thickens and puts pressure on the nerve root or because the tumor itself breaks into the spinal canal to put pressure directly on the spinal cord itself. No treatment is needed unless there is nerve pressure, and then X ray therapy may be effective.

Osteomas (from the Greek *osteon,* or bone) are also benign tumors which occur in parts of the vertebra. The osteoid osteomas grow locally and may produce direct pressure on the cauda equina or the nerve roots and thus cause severe back pain particularly at night, but a pain which is usually relieved by aspirin. Treatment is a matter of radical removal of the tumor and spinal fusion followed by X ray therapy.

Two other benign tumors which may occur are the meningiomas and the neurilemmomas. The meningioma is occasionally seen in the cauda equina, while the neurilemmoma (also called Schwannoma or neurofibroma) arises from the sheath of the spinal nerves. Should either tumor grow and press on the nerves it can cause severe symptoms. The meningioma can virtually be peeled away from the cauda equina, while the neurilemmoma may become quite large before it produces readily recognizable symptoms. Both are best removed under magnification (microsurgery) either with a high-powered magnifying loupe or with an operating microscope.

THE MALIGNANT TUMORS

Sarcomas (from the Greek *sarcos,* or flesh) are extremely rare in the spine. They form less than 1 percent of all bone sarcomas. Many of these tumors (there are a number of forms) are highly malignant but do vary. They usually produce extensive bony destruction within the vertebrae and often lead to collapses of the vertebral body. Occasionally, however, they may result in "ivory vertebrae," in which X rays show just the opposite—a much denser vertebral bone.

With the rapid growth of this malignancy, compression of the cauda equina or its nerve roots almost invariably occurs. Surgery is best limited to biopsy, and X ray therapy is the preferred treatment both to relieve pain and to arrest the rapid progress of the disease.

The other malignancy one thinks of in connection with the spine is the multiple myeloma (from the Greek *myelos,* or marrow) which is formed of the cells of the type normally found in the bone marrow. This tumor usually occurs between the ages of thirty-five and sixty-five and is rarely found in children. It begins with vague and poorly localized low back pain which is often worse when the patient lies in bed at night. In the early stages a diagnosis is rarely made because X rays show little.

Before long, however, the vertebrae are destroyed so that all kinds of vertebral collapse occurs, along with symptoms of nerve root pressure (such as sciatica) from the collapsed vertebra. The character of the pain now changes so that any movement produces much worse pain, and the vertebral bodies may buckle to a point where they are thinner than the disk. There are also blood and urine chemistry changes which help in diagnosis. Surgery is generally contraindicated, but X ray therapy and new drugs may well produce long-lasting improvement.

METASTATIC TUMORS

Metastatic tumors of the spine are one of the most common abnormalities of the bony spine, and almost three-quarters of all spinal tumors are metastatic. The vertebrae are the most common site for tumor metastases, followed by the pelvis, those long bones closest to the primary tumor, and the ribs. It's rare to find metastases to the bones below the knees or beyond the elbows. The cancers with the distinct marked predilection for bone metastases are—most frequently—those of the breast and prostate, followed by those of the lung, kidney and thyroid.

The Institute for Spinal Column Research, in Frankfurt, Germany, routinely removes the entire spinal column for meticulous examination in every autopsy. In 1,000 patients (500 men and 500 women) the institute has shown that 19.6 percent of the men with cancer and 15.6 percent of the women had metastases to their spines. This is thought to happen by way of a complex vertebral venous system whose valves are so built that any increased abdominal pressure, such as in coughing or straining, will reverse the flow of blood and send tumor cells back to the vertebrae. But we still don't understand why, for example, the bladder or uterine cancers don't metastasize to the spine as often as do the prostatic ones.

The frequency of spinal metastatic disease is the reason why it's so important for the doctor to get information on what surgery his patient has had for malignancies. Cancers of the breast, for example, spread to the spine quite long after radical mastectomies, and it's not uncommon to see patients five, seven, ten and even more years after breast surgery who only then developed these metastases.

The pain characteristically is surreptitious in its onset, more often worse at night and only gradually increasing in severity. A sudden pain following little trauma—or even none at all—may be a sign of a pathologic fracture owing to the eating away of the vertebrae by the metastatic cancer. Vaginal and rectal examinations, too, are important here, for many unnecessary spinal biopsies have been done because the physician failed to examine and find the prostatic cancerous nodule or some other rectal mass.

Metastatic cancers may eat away the vertebrae or cause them to become overcalcified (ivorylike in the X rays). In fact, by the time an X ray shows these metastatic diseases a quarter or a third of the bony content of the vertebrae may have been replaced by tumor cells. Biopsies are often in order, and there are various methods, from inserting a special bone biopsy needle for aspirating some of the tumor to doing actual open surgery.

Chemicals in These Diseases

In the diseases covered in this chapter, drugs are of increasing importance. No one need be told of the role of antibiotics in infections; these truly were the miracle drugs of the mid-twentieth century. However, there are increasing limitations for these drugs and increasing numbers of organisms which have developed resistance to the antibiotics and no longer respond as they once did.

Today the new antitumor drugs bid fair to become the next generation of miracle drugs, for a number of malignancies (certain of the leukemias, for example) are reaching the point where we can say we are able to "cure" these cancers with drugs now available. Hormones, too, are being tried, often with considerable success. On the other hand, there are many tumors against which we can do little or nothing with our current chemotherapy (treatment by chemicals or drugs). So drugs are still a matter of success and failure, depending on the particular tumor involved.

Part III

What You Must Know
to Protect Yourself

Chapter 11

HOW TO CHOOSE THE RIGHT DOCTOR FOR THIS PROBLEM

EVERY PHYSICIAN is for one disease and no more . . . the whole country is full of physicians . . . there are physicians of the eyes, others of the head . . . others of the belly, others of the more obscure diseases.

No doubt this sounds familiar, and it isn't too inaccurate a picture of medical practice in today's United States; only it was actually written some 2,500 years ago by Herodotus, the famous Greek Father of History, and he was describing the state of Egyptian medicine of his day. The more things change, it seems, the more they remain the same. And no doubt the Egyptian patients of those ancient days were faced with the same problems of finding the right physician that you are troubled with right now.

But there are ways to approach this as far as low back problems are concerned. There are things you can look for in judging a doctor (whether a family physician or a specialist) which will help you get quality medical care overall, as well as in special problems.

Here are the specific facts you can use to check out the doctor you do find, to assure yourself that he has the proper qualifications. With a physician who fulfills these requirements you can rest comfortably in the knowledge that you and your family are getting the best possible available health care. For the United States does have the finest to offer; it's just that it's a lot harder to find than it was before World War

133

II, and it takes more know-how and skill on your part than it did in those days.

That proper medical care is both important and essential is an elementary observation, but just look at the figures: Every month 750 out of each 1,000 Americans suffer some kind of sickness, 250 of these turn to a physician for help, and 100 are hospitalized. The mythical "average American" consults a doctor four and a half times a year. His needs may involve almost anything: A simple cold or flu or a serious infection may require powerful and dangerous medications; he may require open-heart or spinal surgery or even transplants; his low back problems may range from the nagging constant backache to the condition for which he's carried into a hospital. But what has happened to make Americans feel disillusioned and unhappy about their doctors, and how can you protect yourself?

What Did World War II Do to Medical Care?

Before World War II, medical practice was a different affair altogether; the patients were more comfortable with it and had reason to feel more secure in the care they were given. The real reason was not so much that the doctors were different or knew more but that since the only medical care available was on a much lower and simpler level, the patient could expect the average general practitioner to know all that was then known and to make up for his deficiencies in scientific expertise by a warm personal interest and involvement. The ordinary GP (now almost vanished with the steam engine) could—before World War II—depend on his training in medical school to last him pretty much his whole professional life, with perhaps an occasional postgraduate course and the reading of a medical journal now and again. His knowledge could easily provide his patients with all the benefits of what was then known. Specialists were very much in the minority simply because there wasn't enough medical science to make much difference between the information of the specialist and the GP. Whereas in 1931, 84 percent of physicians in private practice were actually GPs, by 1972 this was turned upside down with 85 percent of physicians now specialists.

Then World War II came with its scientific explosion which swept medicine along with it, and medical knowledge soon became unbelievably vast. With the war, for example, came the antibiotic drugs and the artificial kidney and the "atomic cocktail," with its magic radioisotopes, along with new surgical techniques. We have since added the tranquilizers, the steroids (drugs like cortisone) and medical laboratory tests of a sophistication and complexity undreamed of just thirty years go. Transplants are not even news anymore; open-heart surgery and artificial heart valves and total hip joints are taken for granted by public and professional alike. I could go on indefinitely, but you need no more to see why the specialist is needed today.

Even a good thing, however, can be overdone, and the need today is clearly for more doctors to care for the total patient rather than more of those who care for only one part. When you get a backache from too much gardening the first spring day, if it aches for a day or two, if you apply a little heat or take an aspirin or two and it's gone, you don't need a doctor. But if it lasts, if your low back aches day after day, if the pain is so severe that it interferes with sleep or work or other activities, then whom do you see? What is your best source of help—the specialist or whoever you use for daily health problems?

The Weaknesses of the Specialist

Typical of the weakness of the specialist (I won't go into which field) was the one who treated a man of sixty for intractable low back pain until the doctor finally decided it wasn't in his area and sent the man on to me, a low back specialist. In my questioning of his medical history, the man revealed he had had a prostate operation for cancer two years earlier. Here is the real weakness of the specialist, for I would bet a general practitioner, particularly your regular family one, would have picked up the connection and taken the necessary steps for final diagnosis. In fact, this man was also seen regularly by his prostate surgeon, who also had missed this low back warning of metastases (which is what it was).

It may seem odd that I—a specialist in a specialty, who has fractioned neurosurgery into this new smaller field of the low back—should speak of specialists' shortcomings, but who would know better than one who experienced the difficulties in this problem? All specialists tend to have gun-barrel vision; we see what's in the very center and shut out the periphery, we see the problem, not the patient. And this is not good, for we should see as broad a picture as possible. I try to push myself to do this, and I can tell you it is not easy.

After all, the consultant spends perhaps forty-five minutes, an hour at most, with a new patient. It's very difficult in that short a time to get to know anybody and even harder to define the problem, do the necessary examinations or arrange for whatever tests are called for—and still find time to talk to the patient, to learn about him, what he does, how he lives, what his family and work lives are like, get a picture of his life-style, take a history so that former operations aren't missed. I'm the despair of my secretaries because I will give even two hours just talking to a patient and getting to know him—in short, trying to learn what his family doctor has known for years, and that's why the family doctor is so important.

The Strength of the Family Doctor

A family doctor—the one you and your family have used for years—is your strongest ally and support in getting proper medical care. His concern is for you, and he should give you all the time needed. He will see to it that if a specialist is necessary, you will find your way to the right one. He will be prepared (as we will discuss in the next chapter) to protect you from unnecessary surgery. And after you have consulted a specialist, your doctor will be there to explain what the specialist has found, to discuss any alternatives (even whether you should seek another consultation) and to follow up with any day-to-day care required.

It's the old story: Foot soldiers win wars and hold territory that's been won. Your family doctor is the foot soldier without whom there can be no final victory over disease, no ongoing adequate health care. But in today's complex medical world how can you tell if your family doctor is adequately qualified? It's easy to know if he gives you the time you need, and you can pretty well tell if he's interested in you and if he enjoys doing general practice. If he's interested only in a special field, he may give general medical care only as an unfortunate something he must do to keep up his income, and he will never then do it properly. His lack of interest will show in his reaction to simple routine problems—a headache or backache, your weight and *you* as a person, your family problems. A good test is to see if he really gives you enough time to tell him what's bothering you.

How Do You Know If Your Family Doctor Is Qualified?

The old GPs are gone, there are almost none around (a bare 15 percent of all practicing physicians), and even if they were, you wouldn't be able to get good medical care from them. You need a doctor who knows the medicine of today, and that's asking a lot, believe me.

There are two types of physicians who can fill this bill—the internist and the very new family practicioner (the FP). There are specialty boards which certify doctors as specialists, and they are proof of your doctor's basic qualifications in a particular field, your protection in choosing a physician, evidence that he has undergone a certain amount and type of training which the specialists in his field have determined are needed to be adequately qualified to practice their specialty (anything from, say, neurosurgery to dermatology to pediatrics to radiology or X rays).

The internist has his boards in internal medicine (you can surely see this certificate on his wall because all of us are proud of this evidence of extra work and study and training and display it). He is essentially a specialist in general medicine, for he is trained in all the complex medical (as opposed to surgical or neurological or whatever) problems. He will likely also have some subspecialty, some special interest of his own, such as heart (cardiology) or diabetes (diabetology) or arthritis (rheumatology).

Often, however, the internist, in addition to practicing his subspecialty, will do general practice as well. If you get such a person who meets the previously outlined requirements (interest in general practice, in you and your family, competence), you have found yourself one of the ideal family doctors.

The other ideal, unfortunately, is still a rarity today. These are the board-certified FPs, who unfortunately still number only some 6,000 in the whole country. These are our Space Age GPs, if you will—doctors who are trained in the finest knowledge and techniques of today's medicine but are interested only in doing family practice, what in a simpler world was the old general practice. These doctors specialize, but in family practice, and do only that; in fact, most medical experts agree that these FPs can supply anywhere from 70 to 90 percent of the medical care you and your family will need.

The FP is prepared to handle a great deal of what since World War II has become specialty practice—neurology, dermatology, obstetrics, pediatrics and the like. This would leave only those complicated difficult areas in each field to the specialist, which is as it should be, for it's really a waste of the specialist's time to involve himself—and often overextend himself—with things that are as well and often better handled by the FP.

Checking Your Doctor

It's always ideal if your doctor is on the teaching staff of a medical school, showing that he knows enough to have something worth passing on to young doctors. Next to this is a position on the staff of a hospital which is closely connected with a medical school, and you may find this true today even of hospitals at a considerable distance from medical schools. Certainly as a minimum your doctor should be on the staff of the local hospital, and if there is more than one, it is best if he's on the staff of the largest hospital in your community. Only in these ways can you be reasonably certain that he will have access to the latest things that are being done in medicine, that if you have to be hospitalized, he can continue taking charge of you during your stay there, that he knows the specialists intimately and so can choose the right one for you.

The bigger the hospital and the closer its connection to a medical school, the more medical people are looking over the doctor's shoulder—everyone from nurses to interns to residents, from technicians to other doctors. And let's face it, every one of us does better work when we know there's someone checking on us, watching what we do, inquiring why we do it this way and not another.

The Real Problem with Medicine Today

It may sound strange hearing a specialist extolling the virtues and values of a GP, but I don't think most specialists appreciate how important a good family doctor is to the practice of medicine. The tragedy is that this family doctor is fast disappearing, and that's not good for the public. The trouble lies in the medical schools where the young people, like all students, look up to and emulate their teachers—and in medical schools these are the specialists. If these schools had more family practitioners teaching so that the students had a chance to see what really good general practice is and how important it is, there would be more young doctors going into this essential branch of medicine.

I think the only way may be to require—since so much of medical education is in the last analysis paid for by the federal government, this can be done—that only 10 percent of each class be allowed to go into a specialty. This may well have to be done by law. In Britain, for example, doctors can only go into a specialty if there's an actual need for more specialists so that they have a much better balance. In fact, the people there are protected in more ways than would seem true on the surface, where we might only see that the need for general practitioners is being properly filled. We will see something of the effect of this in medical care in the next chapter.

What Doctor Do You See for That Low Back Problem?

First should be your family doctor, for he knows you and will be aware of many things—what operations you've had, how you function—so he can tell if it's likely to be emotional (he'd know if you've had trouble with your mate or your children, your mother-in-law, your job or whatever). He knows all the things it will take time for the specialist to learn and still not grasp. The generalist also sees you as a total human being, is likely to look for many different things which may be causing the pain or discomfort, whereas the specialist will automatically tend to look only in his own field and really isn't prepared or trained to check your general health.

With the help of your doctor, the two of you can decide together whether you should see a specialist and which one. Even this presents a problem, for there are a number of specialists who could be consulted logically.

What Specialist Should I See for This Low Back?

Involved in low back problems are rheumatologists—arthritis specialists who would be interested in any of the arthritic problems already discussed. Then there are the orthopedic surgeons; they, too, are interested in arthritic conditions, are involved with injuries to the bones and also interested in the muscles, tendons and ligaments, are particularly knowledgeable about the supports such as braces and corsets, but some of them won't operate on the spine or disks.

Next are the neurologists—doctors who specialize in the problems of the nerves, spinal cord and brain. The neurologist is often but not always interested in pain and its diagnosis, but if he is, he's an excellent choice to track down unknown sources of pain. The neurosurgeon, on the other hand, is particularly interested in disk surgery for the low back, in tumors and fractures, and he too may be specially interested in pain and so be an excellent choice. But any particular neurosurgeon may be interested only in brain surgery, so your generalist's advice is important. In any case, the specialist should have his boards in his specialty and the same qualifications in medical school rank or hospital appointments.

It is clear that there are subtleties and shadings of interest, areas which overlap widely and problems—such as osteoporosis—which are likely to fall between two chairs if you try to manage your own case and decide by yourself which specialist you should see with your problem. First, you must know what the problem is (diagnose your own case). Secondly, you must know which specialty deals with this problem to a greater extent than the others. Finally, you must be aware of which specialist is the one most interested and qualified in your particular problem.

It's not an easy problem to solve—which is why I again urge starting with an interested, concerned and well-qualified generalist who is prepared to take full charge of your health care, to direct the chorus of specialists as it were. It's best, of course, always to have a regular family doctor, but if you don't, that low back problem might well be the place and time to start seeking one out.

And If All Else Fails . . .

If you can't get help for your low back problems from any of these sources, you might finally turn either to a low back pain clinic or to a pain clinic. Both these specialty services are increasingly available today. The best way to find either of these specialty clinics is simply to ask your doctor (we keep coming back to this keystone of all medical care). If he can't help you or you don't have a doctor, you could call the nearest medical school or its chief teaching hospital. If you don't have one of these close by, try the largest hospital in your community and gradually go down the line. If necessary, you might try calling a nearby large city, where you are likely to find a range of medical services available.

Somewhere along the way you're bound to find the information you're seeking or reach someone who does know the answer and will have the material at his fingertips.

Getting medical care isn't easy today, but it can be done—if you have the information with which to begin your search and know how to check as you go along.

Chapter 12

OUR TOO-MUCH SURGERY:
How to Know If You Really Need Disk Surgery,
What It Is Like and How Successful, How to
Select Both Surgeon and Hospital

THE EVENING before her operation my patient dashed out of her room, ran down two flights of stairs and locked herself in one of the hospital toilets. It took guards with special keys and tools to bring her out. Another patient began vomiting for no physical reason, trembled and cried a great deal for two days before his surgery. Terrified, these two people wanted desperately to avoid surgery even though they recognized that there was no other way out in either case, that the spinal surgery was essential for their particular problems. While these reactions were extreme, terror actually grips every one of us when we are faced with major surgery. Moreover, one must recognize that hospitals are undergoing a virtual epidemic of infections whose cost is tragically high in lives, in money and in prolonged stays in the hospitals, as well as in their debilitating effects.

Add to this the fact that a certain small percentage (1 to 2 percent is the usual figure mentioned) will die from surgery in general (the anesthetic is commonly the unpredictable and unpreventable cause). This 1 to 2 percent figure includes the fatal accident victim who is rushed into the operating room, the patient with widespread malignancy, the poor-risk cardiac who requires emergency surgery. The mortality statistic for elective lumbar disk surgery is less than 1 in 3,000. All this is still a small price to pay when the other 98 to 99 percent have their lives either saved outright or made livable by these operations. But not all operations are necessary, and objective observers within my own profession agree, as I do, that too much surgery is being done in the United States. Some figures which we will look at in this chapter seem to indicate that virtually half the surgery done in America is unnecessary.

For your own protection it's clearly necessary that you know more about these facts, that you learn how you can make sure that *your* surgery (specifically your disk operation) is necessary; what disk surgery is like and your likelihood of success with it; if a surgeon is properly trained and the ways by which you can judge his competence; how you can judge a hospital, for your life may well depend on the hospital in which you undergo your surgery.

First though a word about this man or woman you deal with, the MD in whose hands you must put your own life and those of your family sooner or later—and probably many times—during the course of an ordinary life.

What Is a Doctor Like?

Doctors really do want to do a good job, try to do their best, but like all human beings, they vary in talent, in interest, in the ability to see themselves objectively and honestly. They are affected by the attitudes of the society about them, by the emphasis on money, by the tendency in the United States to equate competence and success and quality with money and income. But the society—you, the public—must also accept the responsibility for setting many of the standards we all— doctors and patients alike—live by.

Medicine is a hard life, demanding and pressure-filled, for it's not easy to make life-and-death judgments, to take a human being's life in one's hands. Doctors, too, are as affected by fads and trends as the society around us all. The routine removal of children's tonsils and adenoids in the early part of this century was blindly and honestly accepted, and it's only now being seriously questioned in its entirety, yet it would be unfair to condemn those who practiced it in the past.

So, recognizing these facts, let's look at the ways in which you can protect yourself from those surgeons who may be mistaken either through lack of knowledge or from their form of target fixation—and particularly from the relatively few actually dishonest ones like the surgeon whose story of about forty totally unnecessary back operations was recently spread from coast to coast. It's also just as important to protect yourself from the inadequate hospital, for on its facilities and staff your life may well depend should you need surgery.

The Overpractice of Surgery Today

Nobody really knows just how many operations are done every year in the United States; about 14,000,000 were done in 1965, and by now it may well be as many as 20,000,000 or more a year. Both American and foreign surgeons are in general agreement that too much surgery is being performed here today, that our surgeons are too aggressive. There are a number of reasons for this, some clearly shown in the statistics we have. But a simple obvious one lies in the fact that if you train a man for almost two decades of his life (college, medical school, internship and residency, postgraduate work) to do a certain thing, he's going to think in terms of that procedure, is going to try to perform it every chance he gets, will treat his patients in terms of what he's learned and been taught is the right way to attack disease. This is the reason—really a very human and an honest one in most instances—that surgeons think in terms of the medical locker room clichés, "A chance to cut is a chance to cure" and "When in doubt, take it out." After all, if society trains a man to do one thing—whether he be a surgeon or a soldier—he's going to want to fulfill that mission which society has imposed on him. But where society limits the number of medical specialists to those that are really needed—as in Great Britain—then the whole situation is turned around. We will see how this happens shortly.

The problem that we face is a simple one: We just have too many surgeons and too many hospital beds, and the effect is precisely a one-to-one relationship. American surgeons are among the finest in the world, but they're being turned out at a faster rate than our population growth, and with this production rate continuing and population growth slowing down, the disproportion is likely to increase. In October, 1973, the largest group of young surgeons in history received their accolade of recognition as specialists: 1,675 became Fellows of the American College of Surgeons (you can recognize these highly trained specialists by the FACS they put after their names and MDs).

Dr. Guy L. Odom was frank in his 1972 presidential address to the American Association of Neurological Surgeons when he pointed out that neurosurgeons in the United States are at the saturation point. His concern is felt by many of us, with the recognition that any excess in a specialty produces, in Dr. Odom's words, "unnecessary diagnostic and therapeutic procedures." Whereas in 1940 there was a ratio of roughly 1 neurosurgeon to each 1,000,000 Americans, in 1971 this had skyrocketed to 10 such surgeons to each 1,000,000.

In surgery the official voice of the American College of Surgery, *Archives of Surgery,* stated in an editorial in June, 1972, that the production of surgeons—the number of residents in training—is being determined by the selfish interests of the hospitals, which need surgical assistants, rather than any consideration for the "overall need for trained surgeons to serve the community."

The statistics and facts are startling, and one need only turn to studies of the surgical specialty organizations, of Dr. John P. Bunker, the Stanford University professor of anesthesia, and the recent classic study of Dr. Charles E. Lewis, the University of California at Los Angeles professor of preventive medicine. Almost half the young doctors taking residencies (specialty training) are in some area of surgery. There are more neurosurgeons in the state of Massachusetts alone than in all of England and Wales, which have eleven times that state's population. More chest surgeons were certified in this country in 1971 alone than the total number of all such surgeons practicing in England and Wales.

It's becoming clear that the number of operations is determined not by the need for such surgery, but by the numbers of surgeons and hospital beds available. The United States has twice the number of surgeons proportional to the numbers of its people as in England and Wales, and they actually do twice as many operations. But no one has ever suggested that there isn't enough surgery done in Britain.

Dr. Lewis investigated eleven population regions in Kansas for their operation rates, numbers of surgeons and hospital beds. He found that there were three to four times as many operations in some of these areas as in others within the same state for such common procedures (operations which have been fads in surgery) as appendectomies, gallbladder removals, tonsillectomies and hernia repairs. There could be no reason for such vast differences in a relatively small area with a fairly homogeneous population. But Dr. Lewis did find a direct and precise correlation between the number of operations and the number of available surgeons and hospital beds.

All this means is that you had better learn to be careful before undergoing surgery not only since the American surgeon is much more aggressive in his approach to his patients, but also because you are dealing with a highly trained person who is being underused. Being a human being, he will be influenced by a natural and healthy desire to make the most of his knowledge, but he may also be prejudiced in his judgment by these same feelings.

What Is the Quality of American Surgery?

Here, too, we tend to suffer by comparison with Britain. If you take qualifications as the basis for judging the quality of surgery, we suffer by comparison. Virtually all operations in England and Wales (and Sweden, too) are performed by the equivalent of our board-certified or board-eligible physician (a young surgeon who hasn't the necessary years of practice to be awarded his board, although he has the training and other qualifications). But here in the United States almost half the operations done are performed by noncertified surgeons, and the only possible limitation on who can perform operations comes from private agencies, such as the hospitals.

Another problem introduced by the difference in numbers of surgeons is that qualified surgeons in the United States perform only a weekly 3.8 operations (including both major and minor), while in Britain the surgeon does twice that many. About three-quarters of American surgeons spend fewer than nineteen hours a week in the operating room, with virtually one in five putting in fewer than ten hours there. Skill is improved with increased practice and quickly gets rusty and inadequate when it's not sufficiently used.

With all these problems it's increasingly important that you learn to judge the qualifications of both your surgeon and the hospital in which your surgery is to be performed and to learn how to check a surgeon's judgment when he advises surgery.

How You Can Judge Your Surgeon

The fundamental evidence of training and qualifications is board certification. Your surgeon should be both board-certified and an FACS, which you can tell easily, for he's sure to have his certificates on his office wall and his FACS on his stationery as well. In fact, this is a way to double-check your own doctor; the surgeon he recommends should have these evidences of quality except in an emergency or an area with few inhabitants and those widely scattered, as in Alaska or Idaho, when it may not be possible to get such a surgeon. In the average United States community you might well wonder about your own doctor's qualifications if he recommends a surgeon who is *not* board-certified or at the least board-eligible.

It's true that there are some surgeons who are competent, even though they don't have these qualifications, but it's a risky thing to put your life in the hands of such a man. Of course, all the credentials in the world won't tell you about the particular skills of the individual surgeon. But here again a good family doctor won't put his patients in the hands of a surgeon unless he knows this physician has proved his quality over the years.

It's also best to have a surgeon who isn't over sixty-five years of age because surgery is a physically hard life, and it takes its toll. These physicians must be able to stand by the operating table for four or five hours at a stretch while they carefully work away. In any particular instance you will, of course, find exceptions, but your doctor would know this, too, and such an older surgeon will be widely known for his skill and abilities despite his advanced age.

There is one last test of your surgeon. Is he on the staff of a medical school? This is an excellent test, for it tells you what his peers think of his knowledge and competence. But there may be no medical school nearby, or he may not want for some reason or other to be associated with one. Another test is his rank on his hospital staff; high rank in an outstanding hospital is a good recommendation for any surgeon, for good hospitals will only have board-certified or board-eligible doctors on their surgical staff and will be fussy about these, too.

It's also wise to be sure the surgeon works in the field in which you need help. Thus you would want a neurosurgeon to operate on a brain condition and either a neurosurgeon or an orthopedic surgeon operating on your spine or doing your disk operation. Hospital or medical school appointments will quickly tell you this (say, a professor of neurological surgery or orthopedic surgery or whatever).

There is one qualification, of course: that your community may be so small and its hospitals correspondingly so small that it's not possible to support such specialists. In an emergency there's no choice, but if you can wait (and this is commonly so with slipped disks), then your doctor can arrange for your surgery with a qualified specialist at one of the giant centers of medical care, for with air travel today the finest medical centers of the world are within a few hours of your home.

Judging the Hospital and Why

The quality of a hospital shows the quality of its medical staff; good doctors won't associate themselves with poor hospitals, and topflight hospitals insist on high standards for any doctor on their staff. Each one shows the quality of the other and gives an extra dimension by which to check your doctor. Hospitals do vary widely; for example, in New York City, one of the great centers of medical care, a recent survey showed that almost 40 percent of the hospitals should be closed down because such basic requirements as X ray and surgical facilities weren't even "reasonably adequate," as the report put it.

Hospitals in the United States vary as widely as the climate itself and the population. Alaska has five- and ten-bed hospitals, while the great metropolitan medical centers of the continental United States can have 2,000 and more beds. The terms "hospital" and "medical center" are not very meaningful because they are applied at the discretion of the facility itself and can vary from giant 2,000-bed institutions to those of as few as five beds, so ignore the name.

What size hospital should you seek? One guide might be that New York City is setting 400 beds as the minimum size for its hospitals. The reason is simply that smaller hospitals can't support either the staff or the facilities to provide the finest in modern medical and surgical care, except for an occasional special situation, such as the small Kaiser Foundation Hospitals of California or the Hunterdon Medical Center of Flemington, New Jersey. However, much depends on the population of the community and even the area; thinly populated large areas just can't support giant medical centers.

You can get your best care in university teaching hospitals, in the chief hospital of a medical school or hospitals affiliated with medical schools, because they have medical backup with specialists available even in the smallest of the subspecialties. It's easy to check on a hospital; simply look up in your library the American Hospital Association publication *Hospitals*. Each year this magazine puts out an annual guide to the 7,000-odd hospitals in the United States with all the information you need to make an informed estimate of the quality of the institution—how many beds each one has, what services (intensive care units, blood banks, radium therapy and so on) are available. This way, too, you can compare the hospitals in your community and judge both doctors and surgeons.

Chapter 13

X RAYS FOR YOUR BACK:
Myth and Reality, Uses and Abuses

INCREASINGLY the public is alarmed by the stories of tens of thousands of unnecessary deaths from excessive medical X rays, and only recently Ralph Nader and his group have also become involved in this question. Individual horror stories are there aplenty; even highly respected medical magazines such as *Medical Economics* carry reports such as those of one patient whose stomach cancer was missed by a nonradiologist (no X-ray specialist) who took the X rays and another patient who lost both legs when mistreated with X rays by another nonspecialist. Then there's the relatively new medical uses of the terrible atomic bomb. There are the stories about the myelograms, the special X rays used to diagnose slipped disks and other spinal problems, which frighten public and medical profession alike.

Clearly it's essential to get at the facts—to protect you from misuse of X rays and to keep you from anxiety and fear should your doctor feel you need a myelogram.

Radiology: The World of the X Ray

It all really began late on a Friday afternoon in a physicist's laboratory in the University of Würzburg in Germany. It was November 8, 1895, and Professor Wilhelm Conrad Roentgen was experimenting with what was then called a Crookes tube (a cathode-ray tube, father of our own X ray, TV and other imaging tubes). He paid no attention to the fact that he

152

happened to have a screen coated with barium platinocya-
nide lying on a bench nearby. Covering the pear-shaped tube
with black cardboard to test its opacity, he turned on the current in a dark room. Suddenly he noticed a ghostly shimmer-
ing light at a distance. Striking a match, he discovered the
light came from the screen. He knew that it couldn't be due
to cathode rays with which physicists were then familiar, for
he knew these didn't travel this far.

But here was genius at work, for day and night something
now drove Roentgen to work with this strange radiation.
Some brilliant spark led him to recognize this was something
totally new, and he named it *X Strahlen* or unknown rays (X
rays if you will). He soon proved that these rays went right
through paper, a playing card, a book, wood and even thin
sheets of metal other than lead. He discovered the rays cast
an image of the bones of his hand on that original screen.
And on December 22 he took the first medical X ray—of his
wife's hand; it showed her ring and the bones and terrified
the poor woman.

He personally delivered to the secretary of the local Physical Medical Society, on December 28, 1895, his manuscript
"On a New Kind of Rays" for publication. In a few days he
had reprints to which he attached his own X rays and which
he sent to several famous physicists on January 1, 1896.
Probably no other medical discovery was ever put to use as
quickly as Roentgen's rays (it's still often known as roentgenology, roentgen rays and so on). Barely two weeks after
his discovery, medical X rays were being taken and exhibited
in Vienna: a crookedly healed fracture of a finger caused by
a bullet; another utilizing one of the most modern of techniques—injection of a dye to show up arteries on X rays (only
this early one was done on a corpse's hand). During the same
month X rays were being shown in Berlin of a glass splinter
in a hand, in Graz of a needle in a hand and in Vienna of a 6
mm projectile in a hand just before surgery.

It's amazing that in a time of such slow communications,
articles on the uses of X rays in medicine appeared that same

month, January, in New York, British, and Munich medical journals, and in February, in the *Journal of the American Medical Association.* In fact, in January and February X rays were used for every kind of medical purpose, and in February an X ray taken of a bullet in a young man's leg was later filed as evidence in a Canadian court in a suit over the shooting—the first medicolegal use of the X ray.

But all that activity is nothing compared to the heights the use of the X ray has now reached. Just in the period from April through September, 1970, the National Center for Health Statistics reports 180,000,000 visits made for X rays in the United States (112,000,000 for medical and the rest for dental). And 120,000,000 Americans—roughly 7 of every 10 of us—had X rays taken.

Right from the start, in 1896, the reports of X ray injuries began to appear. The earliest victims were the doctors themselves, who developed cancers, particularly of the hands since they exposed themselves without fear to the unsuspectedly deadly rays. Technicians and nurses and even workers in the new industry—all fell victim to the unsuspected killer. In some cases, decades of treatments and dozens of operations with small amputations of the fingers followed by those of hands and arms, all finally ended with death from metastases.

The Menace of X Rays Today

The danger of X rays now—as in the earliest days—is still cancer. But this is the danger of *mis*used X rays, for without this vital diagnostic tool there could be no modern medicine. Latest evidence indicates that the very fetus in the uterus must be protected because those exposed to X rays later reveal an increased cancer risk directly proportional to the numbers of X rays taken of the pregnant mother. Even low levels of radiation can be dangerous.

Dr. Irwin Bross, chief epidemiologist at Buffalo's famed cancer center, Roswell Park Memorial Institute, has discovered that so-called safe levels of X rays aren't all that safe.

The risk of cancer in some children can be increased ten times at the low levels used in pregnant women, so Dr. Bross has called for an immediate revision of X ray dosages—something only a trained radiologist is likely to appreciate and be able to follow in detail.

Actually, insurance companies and the law take their toll of unnecessary X rays. There is, for example, a preemployment X ray examination of the low back being used by industry in the belief that it can indicate the likelihood or danger of future low back problems on the job; only there's considerable evidence this just isn't so.

It's been estimated that as many as a fifth of all X rays are taken for medicolegal reasons. Of fifty-five skull X rays in one study, only one showed anything wrong, according to Dr. Alexander R. Margulis, chairman of the radiology department of the University of California at San Francisco. Another study showed that more than a third of skull X rays are only taken for medicolegal reasons. Perhaps our laws as much as or even more than our medical practices really need marked revision.

In short, the key to safe X rays is the quality of your physician and the knowledge that most X rays should be done by qualified radiologists. These specialists in X rays are prepared to protect you in the taking of the X rays and qualified to interpret or "read," the X rays, which is a complex and difficult business.

What X Rays Are and What They Show

Essentially X rays, or radiographs (once commonly called roentgenographs), work somewhat like the firing of a shotgun through a series of metal rods attached to a wood wall. The metal rods would stop or deflect much of the buckshot, and if you took away the rods, you would see them outlined by the holes made in the exposed wall by the buckshot. Anything which stops the buckshot as the rods did—or the X rays as bone does—casts a kind of negative shadow, an absence of marks.

X rays are actually similar to visible light except that they have a much shorter wavelength. It is even shorter than that of the far ultraviolet rays, but slightly longer than that of the gamma rays given off by radium, which is also part of this same type of electromagnetic radiation. With the high-powered modern equipment, X rays can be generated which are some 250,000,000 or more waves to the inch as compared to 50,000,000 for waves of visible light.

The big plate the radiologist or technician puts behind or beneath you for an X ray is actually a combination of two intensifying screens with the X ray film between. Those X rays which pass through the body strike the intensifying screens; these give off visible light which actually forms 90 percent of the image you see on that X ray film the doctor examines. Where the X rays pass through—the soft tissues of the body—there is light from the intensifying screens to turn the film black, and where the X rays are stopped (by bones, for example), there is no light, so the films remains white. Thus, metal or teeth or bones which stop X rays show up white on the radiograph as does anything else such as special dyes which stop the X rays.

In order to show up soft tissues like blood vessels—or a spinal disk—a radiopaque material or dye must be injected into or around the tissue to stop the X rays. However, it is possible with special radiographic techniques to see much about the brain or spinal cord, for example. If you want to X ray the stomach, you have the patient swallow that despised barium meal which is radiopaque and outlines the stomach since it fills the cavity and presses into each inner wall defect, outlining tumors or ulcers or whatever. Similarly, if you're interested in seeing the blood vessels or brain or lungs or heart, you inject a radiopaque dye to outline whatever you're interested in.

The X Rays of the Spine: Inside and Outside

The plain X ray is the ordinary kind that you're so accustomed to—for a broken finger or a dental examination or the routine chest X ray. The plain X ray of the back is the easiest and most innocuous of the radiographic techniques here, and the most commonly used. Its great virtue is its harmlessness, its safety and the fact that the amount of X ray exposure is not particularly dangerous. It can be helpful in a number of instances in low back dysfunctions, so we always get a plain X ray of the lumbar spine and look at it.

It's a bit of a paradox that while the plain X ray does give us a lot of information, it sometimes gives us too much and sometimes not enough. For radiologists estimate that about one in every four lumbosacral spines that are X-rayed shows some abnormality. The odd thing is that so often the person whose spine shows very obvious and often extreme defects or pathology or anomalies (any deviation from the normal, any abnormality not caused by disease or pathology) will suffer no low back discomfort or symptoms. On the other hand, you frequently find that the person who can barely hobble about because of his back difficulties will have a spine which appears perfectly normal radiographically.

The biggest weakness of the plain X ray is that it reveals very little about the nonbony tissues of the spine. For example, ligaments, tendons and muscles, as well as the disks, show up inadequately on plain X rays. If there is a herniated disk, you can only get slight confirmation of your clinical findings, for all the plain X ray will show is a narrowed disk space.

The big advantage of this technique is its innocuousness. It does, however, show quite well what's happening to the spinal bones—osteoporosis can be seen, and fractures or displacements or malalignments. Osteoarthritis is revealed by the bony spurs which form in this condition. Metastatic and primary tumors, too, can be recognized, but the weakness here is that the metastatic tumors must have destroyed virtually half the vertebral bone before changes show up in the X ray. Infections may also be seen, but they don't become evident until two to six weeks after the appearance of the pain, when presumably the infection is already well under way.

There are, however, special X ray techniques on which we

fall back and which have gained unwarrantedly bad reputations. But first a word about two major developmental anomalies which plain X rays do reveal.

Spondylolysis and Spondylolisthesis

These names are jawbreakers, but if we look at their Greek origins, they will explain themselves. *Spondylos,* as we've noted, is Greek for vertebra, *lysis* means dissolution and *olisthanein* (the "listhesis" comes from this) means to slip. About 4 percent of the population has one of these conditions, but most of these people have neither significant back pain nor disability.

Spondylolysis is a defect (virtually a "natural" fracture) which occurs in the neural arch of the vertebra between the upper and lower facet joints. There is no question about its congenital (present at birth) aspect. It has also been found that in 60 percent of the instances where both mother and father have this condition the children do too. Morever, it is associated with an increased incidence of other congenital spinal defects, such as scoliosis (side-to-side curvature of the spine) and spina bifida in which the bony circle about the spinal cord—the spinal canal—fails to close completely. Spondylolysis is racial in origin, for it appears in 6.4 percent of white Americans, 2.8 percent of black Americans—and 27.4 percent of Eskimo Americans.

However, this condition is never present in the lumbar region at birth, and the youngest child on record with it was a four-month-old. It's believed that this condition develops from stress in people whose vertebrae are structurally weak in this area. Incidentally, this type of defect is never seen in four-legged animals—another price we pay for rearing up on our hind legs. And children with mental and other disabilities which prevent them from assuming the upright posture don't develop either of these two related conditions—spondylolysis or spondylolisthesis.

Most people with spondylolysis never know they have it,

and the diagnosis is made by X rays taken for some other reason. Nothing unusual or different from the normal can otherwise be found, and only occasionally do these patients report some mild low back pain or a generalized ache, pain which may be referred to the buttocks and, most uncommonly, to the back of the thighs. This is rarely enough to incapacitate and is usually relieved by rest, but it is aggravated by such activities as prolonged walking or standing, lengthy auto driving or heavy lifting.

This pain almost always responds to conservative measures, but surgery has been advocated when other help is unavailing. This operation would be either a spinal fusion or cutting out the loose section of bone. When this typically one-sided defect of spondylolysis is on both sides, there may be a separation at the site of the defect, allowing the upper vertebra actually to slip forward. It is this forward displacement which is called spondylolisthesis.

Sometimes no break is necessary, but the condition may result from an abnormally long bony formation between the facet joints which permits the vertebral body to slip forward. A slightly different from normal arrangement of the facet joints, along with a very acute lumbosacral angle, may have the same effect. Congenital formations or degenerative changes may also change the joints so that this same forward movement can take place.

The degree of slippage either from these formations or from a bilateral defect (spondylolysis on both sides of the neural arch) is classified from 1 to 4. In many people the slippage reaches a certain extent and goes no farther, while in others it continues until the lumbar vertebral body slips completely off the sacrum. The fifth lumbar vertebra (L5) is the most common site, although it also happens to L4 and even, rarely, to L3.

Normally the weight of the torso is transmitted in a downward and forward direction so that there is a shearing force exerted between the last lumbar vertebra and the sacrum, but a normal disk between L5 and S1 prevents slippage. With the bony defect of spondylolisthesis the excessive stress thrown on the disk easily produces degeneration. To make matters worse, your muscles compensate for this forward shift, and this in turn increases the stresses on the involved disk.

The postural changes increase stress on ligaments, joints and disks and may result in pain, along with degenerative changes. Since disk herniation may result from all this pressure, the sufferer may also have slipped disk problems with all their attendant discomfort and pain.

Actually I'm often surprised at the large amount of slippage occasionally seen in patients who have no symptoms at all. Careful leading questions in others will bring reports of only occasional mild low back discomfort. The most common symptoms are a generalized aching or low back discomfort aggravated by activity and eased by rest. Prolonged stooping or bending, climbing ladders or lifting make the pain worse. Sciatica, too, occasionally occurs, and—rarely—there may be some weakness of the legs or even some disturbances from either bladder or rectum such as difficulty voiding or constipation.

Spondylolisthesis can usually be handled by conservative measures: avoiding strenuous activities, using mechanically efficient daily activities such as proper lifting postures and general overall back care, such as detailed in the last two chapters. Mild analgesics and sometimes a low back support may help during strenuous activities or periods of pain. But if these don't help and the pain becomes intractable, if the spine continues to slip forward, if the neurological symptoms develop or increase, then surgery may be needed. A number of procedures are being used, essentially aimed at reducing nerve pressures and stabilizing the spine or preventing its further forward slippage at the least.

These conditions can be seen and followed adequately with plain X rays, but if surgery is considered, then more information is needed, and this is when we turn to the myelogram.

Looking Inside the Spine: The Myelogram

It wasn't long after Roentgen discovered he could see bones right through the skin—by the beginning of our century—that greater attention was turned to spinal surgery. The limitations of plain X rays quickly became apparent. In 1918 Dr. Walter E. Dandy (the leading pupil of Harvey Cushing, the greatest neurosurgeon of this century) introduced ventriculography. This technique is still used to make possible X rays of the brain by injecting air into the lumbar spinal canal; this outlines certain spaces that exist naturally in the brain (the cerebral ventricles). But Dandy pointed out that the air also outlined the spinal canal. Within two years others in Norway and Germany—not knowing of Dandy's work—were also using air to show spinal tumors. However, this didn't provide too much contrast and didn't prove too satisfactory for spinal X rays.

In 1922 a material consisting of iodine and poppyseed oil was tried for this same purpose, and it worked. However, the material was like molasses. I still remember how it was both difficult and painful to the patient when we tried to get it out after we had injected it and taken our X rays. But if it was left in the canal, it produced an irritation. It was with relief that we welcomed the use of pantopaque (which was introduced at the end of World War II at the University of Rochester).

An iodine-containing oil, this colorless liquid is injected into the canal. Here it outlines soft and hard structures for the X ray so that we can see, for example, where herniated disk material is squeezing into the canal or where a tumor is growing. Pantopaque is heavier than the spinal canal fluid so that when the patient is tilted in position, the contrast material or dye can be made to run up or down the length of the spine and make it possible to see every section radiographically.

When this is all over, we suction out the pantopaque and can usually get almost all of it out. The British, however, don't usually remove the dye but leave it there. The material is slowly absorbed by the body, the rate depending on the individual so that in some it can be removed by the body itself quickly, while in others it isn't taken out at all. There are newer water-soluble dyes, but these require a spinal anesthetic for their use since they cause pain. These are used widely in Europe and principally in Scandinavia.

If you've been plagued with low back problems for any length of time, you've probably heard about myelograms. Many people are frightened by the terrible stories that are sometimes told, but these are largely mythology, not fact. What we've just described is the myelogram—whether it's air myelography or pantopaque myelography or any other technique. Occasionally a patient does meet up with an unfortunate experience, but with rare exceptions this procedure can be carried out in relatively painless fashion and without complications.

However, myelograms shouldn't be used on a "routine" basis, as are plain X rays. The myelogram is really reserved for those patients who have herniated disks, which don't respond to conservative treatment and where surgery is the next step or those patients who are showing marked neurological symptoms, such as significant weakness from nerve root pressure. It is always used where there is any possibility or likelihood of a tumor, for in these circumstances we want to dot every *i* and cross every *t* in our diagnosis. Finally, we would regard the person with long-standing low back pain which stubbornly refuses to respond to conservative management as a candidate for a myelogram.

The procedure is simple. There's no premedication ordinarily, and you won't even omit any meals. You'll either be sitting or lying down. A little local anesthetic, such as your dentist uses, is injected to numb the area. However, if the patient is allergic to these anesthetics, the procedure is painless enough to be done with only some reassurance, and there's no particular discomfort once the needle penetrates the skin. This is done at the midline of your back roughly a trifle above a line between the height of your hipbones (the iliac crest) which will bring the needle into the L3–4 interspace. A little of the cerebrospinal fluid is collected when the needle has been put into the spinal canal, and then 9 cc of pantopaque is injected.

Now the X rays are taken of the patient in various positions (you are tilted up and down so that the dye runs downhill and outlines the canal from one end to the other). The original needle usually remains in place during the myelogram, and this is now utilized to remove the dye by aspiration. When it's all out, the needle is removed, and the procedure is all over. You'll be kept in bed for twenty-four hours after this procedure and then allowed to go to the bathroom. However, you'll stay as flat as possible and be given lots of fluid for a couple of days more, and then the whole affair is all over.

There is also another newer type of spinal X ray which has particular value in some special instances, especially for the new use of papaya juice, as we shall see in Chapter 16.

The Diskogram

This is the newest of the spinal X ray techniques and more painful than the myelogram. The concept of the diskogram goes back to Dr. Christian G. Schmorl, a German pathologist born at the time of the Civil War. In his painstaking and elaborate studies of autopsied human spines, Schmorl injected the spinal disks with red lead paint to differentiate normal from diseased disks. But not until 1941 did anybody inject a living patient's normal disks with contrast material to make special X rays.

It was 1948 when diskography—the injection of a disk with a dye and its X raying—was first presented as a clinical diagnostic technique by a Swedish investigator. Two years later a pair of Americans at the Cleveland Clinic performed this on three disks which they diagnosed as herniated and were later surgically confirmed. Some use this method frequently and even in place of myelography.

Diskography does produce pain, and you have to be sedated. The pain must be felt so that it can be compared with the back and leg pain bothering you and the problem can be located. It's a matter of placing a long thin needle into the lower three lumbar disks, in most instances, and injecting the contrast material.

The advantages are that the disks themselves can be seen in the X ray, the pain is informative, and there is no reaction to the contrast material, which is completely absorbed within fifteen or twenty minutes. Long-term effects on disks are unknown, and there is the danger it may hasten the normal degenerative changes which take place in disks. But it has given us information on the aging of disks and shown that the majority of patients without symptoms and over the age of thirty-five have X ray evidence of lumbar disk degeneration (as mentioned in Chapter 9).

Diskography is obviously going to become more popular as the use of papaya juice for herniated disks increases. In that new therapy you have to insert a needle into the disk, and as long as you have to do that anyhow, you might as well use it to check the condition of that disk before this new papaya treatment.

Chapter 14

THE ATOMIC BOMB GOES MEDICAL:
Nuclear Medicine and Your Low Back

WHEN AMERICAN scientists opened that terrifying Pandora's box of horrors in July, 1945, they little realized that they were at the same time making possible a new world of medicine which only recently has reached the low back and its problems. For one day that month one of the scientists working at a closely guarded laboratory in the New Mexico desert dropped by a friend's house in nearby Santa Fe and suggested he go to the top of Sandia Mountain that night and look southward: "Before the night is over, you'll know what we've been doing up here."

So it was in the early hours of the morning of July 16, 1945, that the Santa Fe resident saw the brightest flash of light our ancient earth had ever before witnessed—along with the deadly mushroom cloud that marked the coming of age of the nuclear era, the first atomic bomb. But also out of this destructive weapon has come one of medicine's newest fields, nuclear medicine, to fulfill man's ancient dream of the transformation of one element into another. It utilizes the almost-forgotten vision of alchemy to cure disease and to save lives. And now we use this same nuclear medicine for the low back and its problems.

At the heart of our fantastic atomic world lies the tiny atom which makes up all matter. The nucleus, or center core, of the atom consists of two kinds of particles—protons and neutrons—while another type—the electrons—circle around the nucleus much as the earth and planets do about the sun. Like

165

the universe, too, most of the atom is just plain space. If an atom of gold, for example, were enlarged to the size of a bale of cotton weighing 500 pounds, its nucleus would be no larger than a speck of black pepper, but it would weigh 499 3/4 pounds. And in that nucleus is all the fantastic energy of the atom, the power of the atomic bomb.

So far as medicine and our low back interests are concerned, the important word is "isotope." Most chemical elements found in the earth's crust and atmosphere are actually mixtures of isotopes—natural tin, for example, is composed of almost a dozen. Isotopes are forms of the particular element which are identical in chemical properties but differ in the weight of their nuclei. Some of these are stable, while others are radioactive and change with time. These—called radioisotopes—give off alpha, beta and gamma rays until a final stable form is reached. Radioisotopes can be either natural or man-made, and their gamma rays are very close to X rays; in fact, physicists can't tell them apart. It is the gamma rays of radium that have been so widely used medically. Let radium continue to give off its rays. and it will eventually end up as its stable form—lead.

The initial medical payoff of the atomic bomb came on June 14, 1946, when the first shipment of a reactor-produced radioisotope was delivered by the director of research at Oak Ridge National Laboratory, Nobel Prize winner Dr. Eugene Wigner, to a doctor of St. Louis' Barnard Free Skin and Cancer Hospital. That first sample was an almost invisible pinch of white powder, about 1/10,000th of an ounce of a carbon isotope.

The Medical Particles: The "Life" of an Isotope

The statistics and figures of the Atomic Age are difficult to comprehend, but we must. Alpha particles are so small that 100 trillion of them would fit on the head of a pin, and their penetrating power is so slight that a few inches of air or a sheet of paper will stop them. Beta particles are about

1/7,200th as large as the alpha and can travel several yards through air, penetrate barely 1/3 of an inch of human tissue. All of which is important to the use of radioisotopes in medicine, as we shall see.

As the standard of measurement of the rate of decay of radioisotopes, doctors use a figure called a half-life. This is the time it takes for the radioactivity of any particular element to run down, or decay, to half. If an element with a half-life of 10 years starts with 1,000 atoms, there will be only 500 atoms in 10 years, 250 atoms in 20 years, 125 in 30 and so on. But half-lives vary widely from 1 trillion years or more to less than a billionth of a second. The most common radium isotope has a half-life of 1,600 years, but most manmade isotopes in use today have half-lives measured in hours or days at the most. Thus, their radioactivity is gone from the body quickly once they've served their purpose.

Radioactivity and Nuclear Medicine

Don't let the word "radioactivity" frighten you unduly, for the entire world is radioactive, and so are we. There is external radiation background from cosmic rays (charged particles from outer space), and there are naturally radioactive isotopes in the soil and rocks and air about us. We even have an internal radiation background from eating these substances. Finally, as Dr. Norman A. Figerio of the Argonne National Laboratory points out: "A television set, for example, is simply a low voltage X ray machine." Before you run and hide in the closet when your youngster or mate turns on your TV set, however, consider this: a combination of factors, including shielding and your distance from the screen, help make the dosage of radioactivity negligible in almost all instances (only a few months ago some half million color TV sets were found to pose a potential radiation hazard, and the manufacturer was forced by the Food and Drug Administration to institute a corrective program for all outstanding sets). Besides all this, you are constantly exposed to all sorts of unexpected radiation, and usually without harm—bath-tubs glazed with a uranium pigment (they have a lovely yellow color) or even houses built with radioactive stones.

The Medical Radiation-Detecting Devices

It was only in 1955 that almost 5,000 visitors passed through a ten-ton three-inch-thick lead-walled chamber—to stand there for forty seconds while their radioactivity was totaled for those attending an atomic science conference in Geneva, Switzerland. This device is called a whole body counter. It puts a figure on your radioactivity, and it's based on the fact that when gamma rays travel through certain crystals, liquids or plastics, they leave a trail of tiny individual flashes of light in their wake. Medical scientists have put this phenomenon to work to obtain medical information, such as we can now get about certain low back sufferers.

Doctors use whole body counters to study the functioning of the human organism and its systems: to tell how much of the body is fat, and how much lean muscle; to learn about the changes that take place, for example, in the body's potassium in the victims of muscular dystrophy. But where whole body counters tell the total body radioactivity, scanning devices zero in on special organs or areas to "see" inside the body in a very new and special way.

What Nuclear Medicine Really Is

Nuclear medicine has grown to the point where it is now a recognized subspecialty. It came directly out of the atomic bomb because new radioisotopes to fulfill the special needs of this work had to be produced. Dr. Marshall Brucer, the Father of Nuclear Medicine, pointed up this fact when he told how right after World War II there were some 40 radioisotopes but within a few years the number had skyrocketed to more than 1,000, nine-tenths of which were artificial. Radioisotopes are made by putting a chemical element in a nuclear reactor. Now radioisotopes run well into the thousands, and new ones are steadily being added, but medically usable radioisotopes number only in the several hundreds. Only a decade ago it was only the unusual giant medical center which had both the personnel and the equipment for providing nuclear medicine services. Today every good hospital has the capability. This could even be one test you use to determine the adequacy of a hospital (and the doctor and surgeon).

Radioisotopes are put into your body either by something you drink (the famous "atomic cocktail" for thyroid cancer) or by injection. The object is to get to a particular target, the organ or tissue your doctor wants either to examine or to treat. In order to do this, the nuclear medicine specialist uses tracer atoms to tag, or label, certain compounds or tissue—red blood cells, for example, or table salt or vitamins—so that he can follow them and find out, say, what the blood supply to a particular organ is like or how blood vessels are formed, how your body utilizes certain foods or how a transplant is taking. The specialist may use a variety of chemical compounds or elements which have an affinity for the particular tissue or organ he wants to check (heart or bone or lung or brain or whatever).

This works in one of two ways. Radioactive calcium or strontium will find a place in the chemical compounds composing bone and so concentrate there. The isotopes have half-lives of, say, three to six hours, so there is barely time for the medical personnel to prepare the material, inject it or have the patient swallow it, have it reach the target organ or tissue and get the desired information by scanning or the use of a special camera before the radioactivity has burned out.

However, there are radioisotopes such as technetium which have to be attached to some compound which has an affinity for the target organ or tissue desired. In technetium's case it is attached to a complex phosphate which will be taken up by the bone and so is useful in checking your low back for problems we'll discuss shortly.

Another thing the doctors in this field are concerned with is that the particular radioisotopes give off virtually only gamma rays which can be "seen" by the devices used for this purpose. If the material gives off alpha or beta rays, they are of no use in nuclear medicine and can damage surrounding tissues. So there are varied requirements which sharply limit the numbers of medically usable radioisotopes.

In essence, though, nuclear medicine is concerned with the use of radioisotopes in both the diagnosis and the treatment of disease. It consists of putting chemicals into the body—chemicals that continuously transmit what amounts to a radio beacon which can be received and later interpreted by the doctors and their devices. These specialists follow where the isotopes go in the body and how fast, whether they lodge or accumulate there. It's a matter of tracking down chemical reactions (the decaying of the radioactivity) in both space and time simultaneously.

Nuclear medicine is 95 percent or more diagnosis and less than 5 percent therapy. And this is so despite the U.S. Public Health Service survey of five years ago which found that some 250,000 patients with increased thyroid activity had then been treated with radioactive iodine in the United States alone. Nuclear medicine has been one of the fastest-growing specialties in the last decade. In 1970 the nuclear medicine department at Baltimore's Johns Hopkins Hospital was doing some 8,000 patient studies a year (1 out of every 4 patients admitted), and about the same number were being done at New York City's Columbia-Presbyterian Hospital, where they found liver scans the most frequent, with bone the second and chief interest here.

How Nuclear Medicine Looks at Your Spine—and How Safely

For a bone scan a radioisotope examination of your spine, doctors are likely to use one of two chemical elements: either radioactive fluorine (an isotope of the same natural element used to prevent cavities in your teeth) or technetium (a radioactive element artificially produced by bombarding the natural element molybdenum with subatomic particles).

The nuclear medicine physician or technician or nurse will give you an injection of one of these, and you may notice that the source from which they draw the material is as carefully protected as X ray machines so that excessive radiation doesn't escape and do the damage the early unprotected X rays did. The radioactive fluorine will essentially be gone from your body by the time the scan is over, and technetium allows just enough time to be brought and injected into you, for it to travel from the vein to your heart and then to accumulate in your spine. There is no time left for the radiation to do damage to you.

This bone scan will expose you to about a quarter or a third the amount of radiation that a series of plain spinal X rays would. The exposure is in the same ball park as a diagnostic chest X ray, less than a fluoroscopic study of the upper part of your gastrointestinal tract with a barium meal. The injection, too, is innocuous, and there is no possibility of even the rare difficulties or complications as in myelograms.

Two devices are used for seeing inside you in nuclear medicine. First is the scanner, which is an array of radiation counters. Sodium iodide crystals (similar to ordinary table salt or sodium chloride) are each backed up by a photomultiplier tube, all set in a housing which sweeps back and forth slowly above the patient. Each time the device reaches the end of its sweep it moves sidewise an eighth of an inch and then returns so it covers every inch of you before it finishes.

When the gamma rays emitted by the radioisotope strike a sodium iodide crystal, a scintillation, or spark of light, is emitted. The photomultiplier tube converts this light to an electrical impulse which is harnessed in one of a number of ways; typically it trips a hammer which makes a black or gray dot on a piece of paper (sometimes even color dots are used) until an image is formed of these dots. Final interpretation comes from the specialist in nuclear medicine, who works with what is, in a sense, a map of the area or part under study.

Another and newer device is a radioisotope camera which looks not unlike a giant hair dryer and which simply takes a picture of the entire area of radioactivity without the mechanical scanning. This device is a triumph of complex Space Age electronics. It has an oscilloscope face, such as is used to monitor heart attack patients in hospital intensive care units and is not unlike the face of the TV screen. A time exposure of this is made with a still or movie camera so that a permanent record is available for study. The still-camera exposures last from a second to a few minutes, and as many as 700,000 flashes can be recorded in this time. All this information can be handled in any of a number of ways with time-lapse movies as well. Electronic devices may store the information on punch tape or produce computer printouts or any one of many other techniques.

For the patient it's all very simple and trouble-free, but for the specialist it means much study and care to produce his diagnosis.

What Nuclear Medicine Tells Us About the Low Back

Bone scans tell us many things and offer a backup to the X ray which is much more revealing and sensitive than this tool of Roentgen's in picking up certain diseases. One of the weaknesses of X rays is that they won't show changes in the vertebrae until virtually 50 percent of the bone has been replaced by the tumor. But with bone scans we can spot, for example, a metastasis when there has been something in the nature of a 10 percent or so tumor invasion. Thus, when the patient complains of pain in the low back and has a history of surgery for cancer of the prostate or breast, kidney or lung or thyroid, a bone scan is immensely valuable in revealing any metastasis very early. Primary tumors such as the multiple myeloma too are seen much earlier.

A bone scan—simple and innocuous—which is negative or

normal permits us to say with 85 to 90 percent certainty that there is *no* malignancy here. The bone scan can also differentiate between a fresh acute fracture and an old one, can reveal infections or even trauma to the bone which results in hemorrhage directly on the bone's surface. It can also reveal osteoarthritis, rheumatoid arthritis, gouty and psoriatic arthritic involvements of the spine, as well as some glandular dysfunctions of the parathyroids when these affect the bones of the spine.

An interesting area I hope to pursue is the possibility of locating for the first time the microfractures we believe occur in osteoporosis which may be too small to be visualized by X ray and supposedly produce much of the pain its victims report. Certainly the future will bring us many more uses of this powerful and versatile tool for spinal problems.

Chapter 15

LOW BACK SUPPORTS, BRACES AND CORSETS: Use and Misuse

THE USE of low back supports dates far before the beginnings of recorded history. It's almost instinctive for those carrying on hard physical activities to wear heavy leather belts or take advantage of other similar supportive measures. From earliest prehistoric days people learned that splints could give relief from pain, and their use has been an accepted method of treatment since the earliest cultures. In fact, archaeologists have unearthed the remains of primitive man showing evidence of the crude use of splints and braces.

The Edwin Smith Papyrus of 5,000 years ago described wooden splints padded with linen, and splints applied to a fracture of 4,800 years ago have been excavated in Egypt. The papyrus also described how brick supports were molded on an injured person before drying, resulting in something very like body casts, and the ancient Greeks would wrap a clubfoot in bandages impregnated with white of egg dissolved in glycerin, a combination which hardened into the ancient equivalent of a plaster cast. Galen, the great Greek physician of the second century A.D. and founder of experimental physiology, even strapped patients' backs and chests to correct scoliosis.

In the Colorado State Historical Museum in Denver there is a corset made of tree bark; it's split down the front to permit it to be slipped on. This early American back support was made about A.D. 900 in the Indian cliff dwellings of that area. The earliest spinal braces were cumbersome, but in the

174

twelfth century surgeons of the Bolognese school of Italy were already constructing effective spinal supports of relatively simple design and made of both wood and metal.

Ambroise Paré—a rustic barber's apprentice who became one of the greatest surgeons of all times—has been described as the Father of the Art of Bracemaking. Living in the sixteenth century, Paré rose to become surgeon to three French kings, one of whom—Charles IX—saved the Huguenot surgeon from the St. Bartholomew's Day Massacre by hiding him in the royal bedchamber. Besides making the metal corset, leather splints for deformed legs, a hernia truss, artificial limbs and eyes (of gold and silver), Paré devised walking splints. Perhaps he is best known by his modest reply to congratulations on one of his successes: "I dressed him and God healed him."

In the seventeenth century orthopedic appliances improved considerably, and there was a great deal of progress, hastened no doubt by the first governmental intervention in history. For in 1601 England officially accepted responsibility for the disabled with its Poor Relief Act. And in the following century the foundation for modern spinal supports was laid with a broad range of braces and corsets, some of which are still being used, and a variety of materials was utilized even then.

During the nineteenth century in the United States braces were designed for what were then the two widely prevalent diseases of the spine: Pott's disease (tuberculosis of the spine, you will recall) and scoliosis (a side-to-side curvature). Best known was the brace designed by Charles Fayette Taylor during the Civil War when it was called the spinal assistant and incorporated the classic three-point principle of all supports. The Taylor brace pulls the shoulders back.

But the most important brace (the most widely used one today) was that of James Knight in 1884. It was originally meant as a support for spines affected with Pott's disease, and it is often spoken of as the chair back brace. It prevents sidewise or rotary movements, and Knight later modified it for scoliosis, a problem which has been overblamed, particularly for pain.

The Truth About Scoliosis

Scoliosis—the side-to-side curvature of the spine—may arise from a number of causes. It's commonly congenital, but it's not at all unusual to see it occurring as a result of poliomyelitis, cerebral palsy, muscular dystrophy and a host of other diseases of the spine and thorax (the chest).

Whatever the cause, scoliosis has often been unjustly blamed for a variety of low back and other pains. When a doctor sees a person with scoliosis of the low back, he makes a connection in most instances in his own mind between this condition and any pain complaints. But scoliosis clinics (where patients of all ages are seen) find a remarkable lack of low back complaints among their patients. The intervertebral disk at the very apex of the spinal bend has an increased tendency toward degeneration because of the unequal pressure and increased stress on it. Nevertheless, actual statistics reveal surprisingly little increase in the occurrence of low back pain in the long-range studies of people with scoliosis. Furthermore, despite the high incidence of this condition, it doesn't seem to be a major factor in those patients who suffer with low back dysfunctions.

Occasionally, however, the progressive effect of the unequal stress on the back muscles results in a generalized sort of back strain and aching. This is best managed conservatively with a back support and postural exercises. Fusion of the spine is only rarely necessary in the adult. However, when there is a rapid increase in the curvature developing in the spine of a child or teenager, surgery is often indicated.

The Biomechanics of the Low Back

If you were to strip away the muscles from the spine, you would be left with what might be considered a modified elastic rod. This would have an intrinsic stability resulting from the pressure of the spinal disks' nuclei pushing the vertebral bodies apart, while simultaneously the annulus holds the bodies together. If such an isolated spine were maintained in an erect position, the heaviest load it could sustain without buckling would be a mere four or five pounds. This, in fact, is what happens when a person is anesthetized and the muscles are completely relaxed, for the person can't maintain a sitting position by himself since his spine will no longer keep him upright.

Whenever you straighten up from a bent-over position, you're utilizing the lumbosacral spine as a fulcrum and throwing a force of more than a quarter of a ton onto the lower lumbar and the sacral regions. Every time you lift an object from a bent-over position the weight of that object becomes multiplied by a leverage factor of 12 to 16 times, depending on the length of your torso and the position of your arms (how far the object is from your body, for example). Thus, the frail woman who leans forward to pick up her tiny child can throw a strain of as much as half a ton or more onto her lumbosacral spine.

If you notice your torso the next time you try to lift something very heavy (and it's true of all strenuous activities), you'll realize that as you strain, all the abdominal and chest muscles tighten, and you can even feel the pressure in your abdomen and chest. In short, you actually increase the pres-

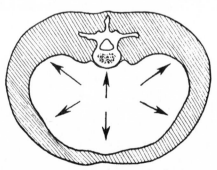

Figure 10. Abdominal.

sures inside both abdominal and thoracic cavities (the so-called intercavitary pressures). This in turn converts the entire trunk into a fairly rigid cylinder and reduces the load on the low lumbar spine by at least 30 percent and on the thoracic spine by 50 percent. Utilizing this principle, the load on the lumbar spine can also be markedly reduced by the wearing of a tight abdominal corset, but you pay a price for this.

The Role—and the Danger—of Low Back Supports

Of importance to your care is a recently done study of the electrical activity of the trunk muscles during lifting, for the amount of this electrical activity can be used to gauge the force and amount of muscular contraction. It was shown that both muscle contraction and intercavitary pressure increased in proportion to the size of the load lifted. But—and this is the important finding—when the patient wore a corset which provided abdominal compression, the electrical activity of the abdominal muscles markedly decreased—clear evidence of reduced muscle utilization and function with external support.

Thus, the use of an abdominal corset or other support will result in reduced muscle use and, if prolonged, can end in muscle atrophy. Clearly, if an abdominal or other external support is to be used regularly, the wearer must compensate with intensive abdominal and postural muscle exercises to keep all trunk muscles in good condition to prevent atrophy. Under all ordinary circumstances a low back support should be considered only a temporary expedient for anyone with low back problems—something to be supplanted as soon as possible by strengthened abdominal and trunk muscles.

Spinal Supports: Purposes, Fact and Fancy

A back support is intended to accomplish three things. First, it should limit the amount of spinal motion in any particular way (keep you from bending forward or backward, twisting or whatever). Secondly, it should correct posture, usually by either reducing the spinal curvatures or making you hold your torso in a different posture. Thirdly, it should reduce the mechanical stress on the lower lumbar spine by providing abdominal support, by limiting the degree of motion of the lumbar spine or in other ways.

Any spinal support exerts some immobilizing effect on the part of the spine it contains. However, study has shown that motion then tends to be increased in the spinal sections adjacent to the ends of the appliance. There is increased lumbosacral motion in some people when a long spinal brace is worn, and so a brace used after a lumbosacral fusion may actually increase motion where immobilization is being sought—a matter of fact over fancy. The design and selection of a spinal support are something for a highly trained doctor to prescribe.

Brace vs. Corset—and Some Tips on Wearing Them

A brace differs from a corset only in that it has horizontal rigid elements; in all other respects they are similar. Corsets may also be made fairly rigid by the addition of steel bars running alongside the spine. Sometimes brace and corset are combined in a single design to gain the best of both worlds.

The advantages of a brace are that it limits motion to a greater degree. It also gives better lumbar positional control, and it limits lateral and rotary motion as well.

The corset, on the other hand, has advantages, too. It's more acceptable, particularly to women, from a cosmetic point of view because it's less conspicuous. It gives better control over obesity and is better for the overweight patient. Moreover, the corset is lighter than the brace, and its long-term use is thought by some to be less likely to weaken the muscles. It's often more acceptable to the elderly, and finally, it's more likely to give abdominal compression.

Today's low friction materials have made all these appliances more comfortable to wear, and you can further help by wearing the device over some clothing. Moisture makes the rubbing worse, and this can be minimized with perforated or absorbent materials. You should ask for detailed instructions on how to put on and remove the appliance and how to care for and clean it.

THE BRACES

Braces to support the lumbar spine are based on a three-point pressure principle. The supporting pressures must come from three directions. For example, there may be a backward thrust against the front of the hipbones or pelvis; a backward pressure against the rib cage, the front of the chest; and a forward thrust against the low back and lumbar spine.

The specific location of these three points may vary. In the Williams lordosis brace, for example, the components are reversed in that there are two pressure points at the back; the low thoracic spine and the sacral region oppose the single front force at the lower abdomen. In all cases, however, the sum of the two points in one direction should be equal to the opposing single one, which should be roughly midway between the two opposing ones.

A recent survey of about 2,000 orthopedic surgeons found that 54 percent preferred Knight's spinal brace, and 19 percent the Williams brace, while the next most frequently mentioned was a bare 5 percent. To give you an idea of what braces are like, let's look at Knight's spinal brace, which was first designed 100 years ago. There are two horizontal bars reaching across the back from side to side; the upper one is about the level of the diaphragm, while the lower one is at the level of the hip joint. Two vertical bars connect the horizontal ones and follow the curve of the body along its side, while two others run parallel and at each side of the spinal column. These are usually covered with leather. There is a center oblong pad whose width is about half the distance from side bar to side bar across the abdomen. This pad is set right in the center of that expanse, with three straps on each

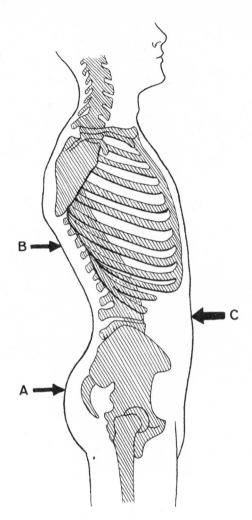

Figure 11. Diagrammatic illustration of the "three-point pressure" principle in design of the Williams lordosis brace.

side for taking the appliance apart and putting it on, and is adjustable so it can be tightened in place. With modern strong lightweight metals, the whole thing is surprisingly

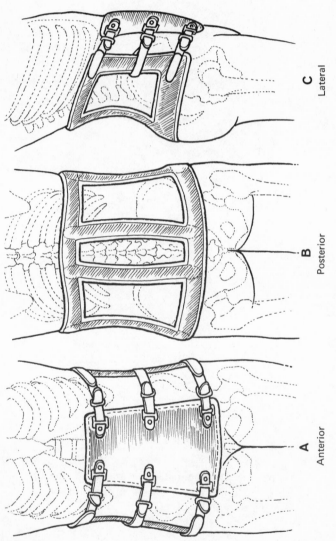

Figure 12. The Knight spinal brace.

A
Anterior

B
Posterior

C
Lateral

light. It limits the wearer's freedom of motion in bending, while providing abdominal compression.

The other braces are designed in a host of different ways with most, like the Knight brace, supportive in nature, although the Williams lordosis brace is designed to put constant corrective pressure onto the lumbar spine and so to reduce the spinal curvature.

THE CORSETS

These are constructed of fabric reinforced with flexible or rigid stays and adjusted by side or back lacing. Side lacing gives firmer back support and makes possible heavy steel bars in the back for contouring and reinforcement. One type of corset is the trochanter belt which circles the hips like the bottom half of a bikini swimsuit. These can be anywhere from one to three inches in width, and they support the sacroiliac joints; such an appliance or a similarly fitting snug leather belt has long been worn by heavy laborers.

Corsets can be large extensive appliances which cover from the lower end of the chest down over buttocks and hips. Termed lumbosacral corsets, these are the most commonly used of all appliances and often have steel bars in the back parallel to the spine.

The Rarer Supports

Less frequently used are supports of leather, plaster of paris or even plastic materials. These have the advantages of precise fit, the widest distribution of pressure and lightness. While plastic supports are very easy to clean, they are also quite expensive. The molded leather jacket, however, absorbs perspiration and is hard to clean.

Plastic jackets are chiefly used in those instances where the support will be needed permanently, whereas the plaster of paris ones are often used for short periods since they provide an accurate fit and a rigid device at low cost.

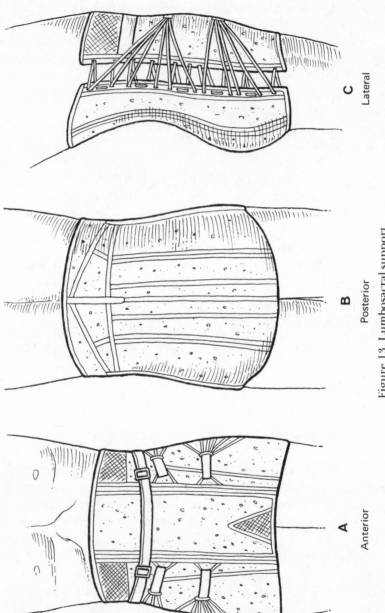

Figure 13. Lumbosacral support.

A
Anterior

B
Posterior

C
Lateral

The Danger of the Low Back Support

The only real danger is psychological dependence on the device so that its use becomes permanent with resulting atrophy of the trunk muscles instead of being used to give the person a chance to build up his own muscles and posture to do the job. Except in special instances, low back supports should be only temporary, just a single first step on the road to full recovery from low back dysfunction.

Part IV

The Answers to Your
Low Back Problems

Chapter 16

PAPAYA JUICE AND RABBITS' EARS:
Will They Make Surgery Obsolete?

THE FRUIT is exotic and tropical and demanding, rewarding to the people who have long known its uses. Only it took a rabbit's ears to reveal the promise of this fruit's juice to low back sufferers, for more than three-quarters of the nearly 10,000 people who have come under the influence of this fruit have been helped. It's all strange and fascinating and excitingly hopeful for you, so here is the story of the papaya and its juice.

The Magic Papaya

It's more a large plant than a tree, for despite the fact that it sometimes reaches twenty-five feet, it's not as woody as a tree should be and usually is. This small tree or large plant bears the name *Carica papaya,* and its origin is unclear, for it may well be the result of a blending of several varieties of Central American *Carica* plants. The papaya tree is cultivated throughout the tropics, where its potentials have long been known and utilized. The local inhabitants commonly wrap any tough meat in papaya leaves overnight or rub the meat with the juice of the plant or its fruit. It does make the meat more tender, and in this strange property lies the magic of the plant.

The tree is usually grown from seeds and produces its first fruit before it's a year old. This papaya fruit is large and not unlike a round or elongated melon, has flesh of an orange or deep-yellow color, juicy and somewhat sweet. It's eaten as a popular breakfast fruit in many tropical countries, is served in salads or cooked in a variety of deserts or as a vegetable. But the plant does require a warm climate, and any heavy frost quickly kills it.

It's in the unripe fruit, in the stem and the leaves of this plant, that the milky juice with its magic protein-digesting ferment, or enzyme called papain, can be found. This ferment is remarkably similar to the digestive enzyme pepsin, which the stomach puts out to break down the proteins in food (such a ferment is termed a proteolytic enzyme). The milky juice is usually obtained by putting small, shallow cuts in the muskmelonlike fruit, while it's right on the plant. From these scratches oozes the milky juice, and when this has hardened into a semisolid or solid mass, it's scraped off. This material—dried and powdered—has for a long time been used as a source of papain and is sold in a variety of preparations for indigestion or simply as the chief active agent in meat tenderizers.

How Meat Tenderizer Works

For almost 250 years it has been known that the stomach juices will dissolve chunks of meat, but only relatively recently have we recognized that all life—the living cell itself—is really just a series of chemical reactions, most of which are controlled by ferments. Besides all this, the digestion of food depends on these enzymes.

Digestive ferments start working on food right with the saliva that moistens everything in the mouth. Take the proteins you swallow. The enzyme pepsin in your stomach has a difficult job to do: It must take large complex insoluble protein molecules and convert them to much smaller, simpler and water-soluble molecules so that these can be absorbed and sent off in the bloodstream to reach the organs and tissues of the body where nutrients are needed to keep the life processes going.

These enzymes of the animal world—of your stomach and mine—are not the only ones nature has developed to do this job. In plants, too, there are proteolytic enzymes to reduce the size of protein molecules so that these can be readily used by the organism. This is what papain is and does. Any meat you treat with it becomes meat that has been partially digested for you; because these first steps have been taken, the meat you then eat is more tender, more easily digestible.

This information struck two investigators at the same time: that somehow an enzyme which broke down protein—specifically fibrocartilage—might somehow influence the strange process which produces the symptoms of disk disease and causes disk degeneration. All this on top of the strange flopping of rabbits' ears have opened a new hope for the terrible slipped disk within barely the last ten years.

Chymopapain, Chemonucleolysis and Rabbits' Ears

It all began with an article in the *Journal of Experimental Medicine* in 1956. Dr. Lewis Thomas had been injecting proteolytic enzymes into the veins of adolescent rabbits in connection with some research he was conducting on blood proteins. But one day, twenty-four hours after he'd started these injections with papain, the rabbits' ears began to hang down like those of spaniels! Careful study revealed that the papain affected all the cartilaginous tissues of the rabbit and broke down one of its constituent proteins (chondromucoprotein, which is also important in the intervertebral disk). The cartilage cells were not injured, and within forty-eight hours the rabbits' ears were perking right up again. Moreover, there was no effect on any other tissues in the body. And it was all reported in that 1956 article in this somewhat formidable-sounding journal.

With this Dr. Carl Hirsch began doing some thinking. In 1959 he published an article on the pathology of low back pain and suggested the possibility that a cartilage-dissolving enzyme injected into a spinal disk might help disk disease.

Dr. Lyman Smith of Elgin, Illinois, had also noticed Lewis Thomas' remarks on papain. The work now began in earnest, and crude papain was soon discovered to have a powerful action on the spinal disks of rabbits.

A variety of proteolytic enzymes were tried out, and chymopapain (an enzyme from the papaya which curdles milk) was chosen since it had a strong effect on the intervertebral disks and the lowest level of tissue toxicity. It was discovered that injecting as little as a hundredth of a milligram (a milligram is 0.015 grains) into an intervertebral disk completely dissolved the nucleus pulposus in adolescent rabbits. With dogs it took a tenth to a half milligram to do the same. With these discoveries the doctors were soon working excitedly in a new assault on the problem of herniated disks.

The work now concentrated on dogs, and a narrowing of the injected disk spaces could be seen in X rays as early as seven days after the chymopapain was used. With smaller doses, the disk would be completely reconstituted two years later, shown by X ray, microscopic and gross examinations. With doses 10 or even 100 times the effective ones there was a permanent effect on the disk. However, all these tests were on the normal disks of healthy experimental animals.

The dachshund, though, commonly suffers a slipped disk. As mentioned earlier, this dog is similar in its hereditary defects to the achondroplastic human dwarf and so is one of a few animals that also suffer these spinal problems. In fact, the dachshund often becomes paraplegic from a herniated lower thoracic or upper lumbar disk. So this dog proved an ideal experimental animal for testing chymopapain. The results were excitingly satisfactory.

All the tests seemed to ring true, including trials of chymopapain's safety under many different circumstances. Nerves were bathed in solutions of the enzyme or injected with it. The chemical was injected into the veins of the animals and produced no significant changes in blood pressure or heart rate or other important characteristics. Only when the dosage was raised to 20 to 200 times the amount needed for the disk was there any serious toxicity.

The stage was now set for the final experimental use of this material on humans. And here, too, it has proved out, according to most investigators and the only official medical body which has investigated it on any meaningful scale.

Chemonucleolysis and Chymopapain Come to People

Only after all this preliminary work did Dr. Lyman Smith finally begin injecting human patients in July, 1963, and his first published report on ten patients appeared the following year in the *Journal of the American Medical Association.* With his report of the first seventy-five patients in 1967 in the prestigious *Journal of Bone and Joint Surgery,* interest grew in what has come to be called chemonucleolysis (meaning a chemical dissolution of the nucleus pulposus). There are now about fifty investigators—mostly orthopedic surgeons with a half dozen neurosurgeons—working with chymopapain, and the number is steadily growing as the results continue to prove successful.

How Chymopapain Relieves the Pain

This is the $64 question. Only we really don't know the answer. Something happens when this enzyme is injected into the degenerated or herniated disk. However, some experiments indicate that there is some biochemical mechanism at work which does provide pain relief. The chymopapain acts selectively and specifically by dissolving only the central portion of the disk (the nucleus pulposus) with little effect on the outer fibrous ring of the disk (annulus fibrosis).

It may be that chymopapain interferes with the water-binding properties of the disk's chondromucoprotein, which it attacks. This would explain how the ferment can produce the rapid relief of the pain we see in many instances. It would also explain why there is an actual reduction in the extrusion of the disk we see if we do surgery on them after an injection of chymopapain. Finally, it explains why there is a marked narrowing of the intervertebral space as we can see in X rays taken shortly after the injection. This reduction remains present for many years.

Our Experiences with Chymopapain

The American Academy of Orthopaedic Surgeons—the specialty organization of orthopedists—has only recently published its *Report of the Committee on Chymopapain,* the latest and most definitive statement to date on this exciting new approach, this chemosurgery (surgery by chemicals, not by knife). And the results seem to me to be pretty conclusive, as was this report.

On September 14 and 15, 1973, each of the approved investigators (the drug at this time can only be obtained for human use with the approval of the Food and Drug Administration) appeared at a conference held by the Committee on Chymopapain. Each presented his own experiences with the enzyme.

A total of nearly 10,000 patients had been given injections of chymopapain for low back pain with or without sciatica; these were sufferers who had failed to obtain relief from a period of conservative treatment, and only those who were regarded as candidates for surgery were given the enzyme injections. Of this overall number more than 8,000 had been followed long enough for the committee to believe it was on solid ground in doing an early result evaluation.

Of almost 7,000 patients who had undergone neither previous surgery nor injections of the enzyme, 86 percent were improved—72 percent markedly so and 14 percent slightly. Of the somewhat more than 1,000 who had already had unsuccessful surgery, 71 percent were improved—more than 54 percent markedly so and almost 20 percent slightly.

There was another interesting finding in 262 patients who

underwent surgery when chymopapain couldn't help their pain. Of these only 11 percent proved to have had extruded fragments of disk when the surgery was performed; the rest had very slightly bulging disks or nothing wrong at all. Clearly, more than disk herniation was causing the pain in many of these patients, and so chymopapain couldn't be blamed for its failure to help them. All of which emphasizes once more the fact that we really don't fully know what causes the pain in disk disease.

There were a number of other results which you may find of interest for yourself or someone close if either of you should suffer with a disk problem. Some of the investigators injected one disk, some did two and some even three. The results were pretty close, but the two-disk injections seemed to give a little better results, although the differences were probably of no real significance. However, it would seem that when a larger amount of the enzyme is injected, somewhat better results were achieved. The results were also checked in relationship to age: While somewhat better percentages in the way of marked improvements were achieved in the fifteen- to nineteen-year-olds and the sixty to eighty-nine, the figures are probably not meaningful, and there is little real difference in the results obtained with different age groups.

Complications and Contraindications

The most frequent and serious complication arises as a result of the fact that chymopapain produces sensitivity. Since about 1 percent of the population is allergic to the enzyme, a second injection is now prohibited. However, some patients who got a good result but afterward had a recurrence located other investigators; not telling of their first chymopapain, they were given a second injection. Of the fifteen known instances, marked relief was obtained in thirteen, and only one had an acute anaphylactic reaction.

This most frequent complication is anaphylactic shock, a

violent reaction to an injection of any foreign protein such as chymopapain—a sort of " immediate allergy." With this reaction there is a sudden collapse, and the blood pressure drops precipitously (owing to dilation of the small blood vessels), there is extreme difficulty in breathing (owing to muscular spasms severely narrowing the lung's air passages) and the skin takes on a bluish tinge, while there may also be intense itching, particularly about the face.

Treatment of anaphylactic shock is aimed to restore normal blood pressure and maintain breathing. Epinephrine, or adrenaline, is most effective here, but recovery from this shock is sometimes spontaneous. Antihistamines and the steroids are useful only for controlling the minor symptoms, such as itching. Several patients have been reported going into anaphylactic shock, and one proved to be a person who only afterward admitted to a previously known allergy to Adolph's meat tenderizer, which contains papain.

Other complications have occurred, but these are really rarities—with one instance or so of each type—or are fundamentally unrelated to the chymopapain itself, such as a fractured rib or a disk infection. Moreover, one should only compare any problems that arise from chemonucleosis with the other alternatives for these patients, and unless the patient is a candidate for surgery, he shouldn't be considered for chymopapain. In short, we must compare any ill effects or complications from chymopapain with those that might and do result from surgery.

The committee found 55 anaphylactic reactions with a single death in the nearly 10,000 reported uses. There were also 22 delayed reactions—hives or urticaria—which appeared some days after the injection. Other reactions included some patients with thrombophlebitis and disk and other infections. Painful muscle spasm is frequently seen, sometimes along with a headache, but these don't last very long.

The contraindications are simple and obvious: pregnancy (we don't like to give anything not absolutely necessary at this time); allergy to meat tenderizer or papain; a normal disko-gram; a prior chymopapain injection; and certain other specific problems (spinal tumor, progressive paralysis and a few similar things).

What Is This Injection Like and What Happens?

All but one of the investigators routinely perform a disko-gram, and most use myelograms to study the patient beforehand. Almost all the investigators use a general anesthetic and do the injection in a special hospital room for the purpose. A few use a local anesthetic, and a few do it in an operating room.

It usually takes three-quarters of an hour to an hour from the start of the anesthesia until the injection is finished, although some doctors do it all in twenty or thirty minutes. The average hospital stay is some six days, and a frequent complaint after injection is back pain or severe muscle spasm which usually lasts only a few days.

Some patients achieve dramatic recoveries with their nerve root pain gone almost immediately, some even waking up in the recovery room with their sciatica relieved. On the other hand, there are patients who report a feeling of insecurity, and a few doctors prescribe a back support until the sensation is past, usually within some six weeks. Spinal fusion was performed on 15 of the nearly 10,000 injected.

Going back to work depends mostly on the person and the type of work. Sedentary workers can start as soon as the soreness and discomfort are gone, usually some two or three weeks later. The heavy manual laborers don't go back to work for four to six weeks, and some may not for as much as four to six months after injection.

Final decision on success or failure with chemonucleolysis shouldn't be made for at least a year simply because some of the patients keep improving steadily as time passes. The comparison with disk surgery is in a sense a matter of simply how long each one interferes with normal life patterns, and one investigator has reported finding that patients with chymopapain return to work in about a third the time his disk surgery patients take. At least six weeks should be allowed to pass with no improvement before chymopapain can be considered a failure and disk surgery resorted to.

The Conclusion About Papaya Juice

The Committee on Chymopapain of the American Academy of Orthopaedic Surgeons concludes with the recommendation that the injection of chymopapain is "an acceptable . . . and effective method of treatment of pain resulting from an abnormal lumbar disc . . . " and agree that it is safe so far as any reasonable medical probability is concerned. However, there is still argument between two groups of specialists both involved in disk surgery and this area.

The Neurosurgeons vs. the Orthopedic Surgeons: Why?

The neurosurgeons as a group are opposed to the use of chymopapain, and the orthopedic surgeons, as we have seen, like it. My own feeling—and the head of the FDA's drug bureau, Dr. J. Richard Crout, has only recently been quoted in *Medical World News* in a similar vein—is that the "controversy" is a matter of groups with different interests.

As a group the neurosurgeons oppose chymopapain, but to the neurosurgeons lumbar disk disease is their bread-and-butter surgery. As we've already seen, they do a lot of it, and they also make their living at it. So if chymopapain is successful, it will cut out a lot of their work.

But many of the orthopedic surgeons don't do disk surgery because they may not be as well trained in back surgery. In fact, they may sometimes be a little nervous about it, for it does get a little hairy at times. But they wouldn't hesitate to do chymopapain injections. So there is also an economic factor at work here in some of the attacks on chemonucleolysis.

The enthusiastic reports on this method of treating disk disease were based on its use by a small group of physicians who pioneered the technique. Because chymopapain is a controversial drug, before the U.S. Food and Drug Administration was willing to approve this substance it established what is called "double-blind placebo controlled trials" in December, 1974. This means that vials of medicine which were supplied to the research physicians contained either chymopapain or a placebo (a harmless substance which produced no particular action). The term "double-blind" means that neither the doctor who performs the injection nor the patient is aware of the true nature of the injected substance. When this study was reviewed by the FDA on July 15, 1975, all the investigators were surprised that the clinical results of injecting chymopapain and the placebo were nearly identical. It appears obvious that additional research is necessary before the final word on the effectiveness of chymopapain is forthcoming.

My Own Feeling About Chymopapain

I believe that when everything has been tried—bed rest, back supports, exercises, medication, the whole conservative approach—and nothing gives the patient relief from his pain, the next step might well be chymopapain before any actual cutting is done. It's still experimental, but there's a large body of success to speak for it, and I look forward to its future.

Chapter 17

ACUPUNCTURE AND ALPHA, MANIPULATION AND CHIROPRACTIC: For Your Aching Back?

THIS IS a story of the Stone Age and the Space Age; of medical practices that work, but we don't know why; of America's grand old man of medicine, the late Dr. Paul Dudley White, and his amazing research of a half century ago; of the ancient Orient and America's now generation in both medicine and the public; and—most of all—of what all this has to offer for your aching back, how it can help—and how it can kill.

For this chapter is the story of the role of acupuncture, its uses and its dangers; of biofeedback—alpha—and what it is doing and how it is now suspect; of manipulation and what you really can expect from it; and of what we know about chiropractic.

Probably the single hottest interest today is in the needles, in acupuncture, one of the oldest therapies we know of. I first learned about acupuncture when I served in the Army in Korea. That was long before the United States had become interested in this ancient Oriental medical practice. It was 1950, and a young Korean attached to our Army was a sort of houseboy around the officers' quarters where I lived. When drafted, the young man had been training to become an acupuncturist, as his father was, and I spent considerable time with him learning about his techniques. However, in Korea, acupuncture was then looked down upon by the trained physicians as a matter of superstitious practices limited to the peasantry, the countryside and the uneducated.

The upper and educated classes in the cities used Western types of physicians and medical care.

However, when I was transferred to Japan after the active fighting in Korea was over, I found a different picture. In Japan acupuncture was used by many of the most educated and the leaders in every field. The acupuncturists specialized in particular problems, were well trained and seemed to get results; at any rate they certainly satisfied their patients, who often returned for help with their medical problems.

Acupuncture: Theory and Fad

Acupuncture seemingly goes back to the Stone Age, for there are stone needles that have been preserved, but at the very least it is 5,000 years old. What is overlooked is that acupuncture is traditionally a metaphysical treatment based on the concept that the body corresponds in a variety of ways to both the universe and the body politic, the state. Then there is the concept of yang and yin, whose constant struggle both in nature and in man determines health or disease in the body. Yang is the southern side of a mountain—the male force or positive, light and warm—while yin is the northern side of the mountain—the female force or negative, cold and dark. The body organs too are divided into the yang ("working" or "active"—stomach, urinary bladder, large intestine and so on) and the yin ("storage" or "passive"—lungs, heart, spleen and the like). In short, the theory does lose all contact with any experimental or scientific fact.

The theoretical basis for acupuncture is that when these yang and yin forces are in balance, the person is healthy; when this equilibrium is upset, the individual is sick. The needles are used to allow the excessive force to escape and so to restore the balance and, with it, health. The numbers of the acupuncture points vary according to the authority: Some describe 295 points, and others 365; there are those who mention points numbering in the 600s and 700s; some even talk of more than 1,000. The points for any particular body organ are connected by invisible channels through which the yang and the yin assist the *chi*, or vital energy, to circulate; these canals are the meridians, or *ching*, each of which is connected to an important organ.

Acupuncture, always widely practiced in China, was actually introduced into Europe by a Dutch surgeon as long ago as the end of the seventeenth century and has had many adherents there up to today. Yet it never took hold in the United States until the New York *Times'* James Reston reported his personal experiences with this ancient therapy a few years ago. He told of relief from his discomfort after an appendectomy. But Western physicians have long known that reassurance and even sugar pills—placebos—can and do make patients more comfortable after surgery.

In any case, acupuncture soon became a fad and swept the country as widely as did the Hong Kong flu only a few years ago. In a nationwide survey the well-known medical magazine *Medical World News,* in its July 19, 1974, issue, reported a West Coast acupuncture venture with six clinics which had already treated more than 15,000 patients and was planning two more clinics and estimates of several hundred to several thousand doctors practicing acupuncture in California. *Medical World News* found that Washington, D.C., had a total of thirteen acupuncture clinics, one of which has a staff of 60 and a record of having already treated more than 6,000 patients. And one Northeastern clinic is treating 100 to 120 patients a day.

The treatments are for everything from obesity to sexual impotency, from alcoholism to osteoarthritis, from insomnia to you-name-it. But make no mistake, these treatments don't come cheaply, for they run as high as $100 a treatment with an average, *Medical World News* found, of $20 a treatment after the initial $50 charge.

Up to a very few months ago too much of the information on acupuncture has been from those who either had material reasons for pushing the technique or were biased for a variety of reasons. Now, however, for the first time we have some trained scientific observations available, two careful studies by one expert, along with some medical reports from that hot bed of acupuncture Washington, D.C.

THE FACTS ABOUT ACUPUNCTURE: FROM CHINA AND THE UNITED STATES

Dr. John J. Bonica, America's leading authority on pain and professor of anesthesiology at Seattle's University of Washington, spent three weeks in China in 1973 as a member of the first official American medical delegation to vi' t China. He visited five medical schools, fourteen hospitals, three research institutes and a health spa, along with some fifteen cities, communities and industrial facilities. Besides this, he was in touch with other physicians who had visited China and studied the literature on the therapeutic acupuncture, and he reported it all in the *Journal of the American Medical Association (JAMA)*.

He found that the acupuncture points used varied widely from one hospital to another, that as a means of anesthesia the use of acupuncture is far from the many and exaggerated claims. For a period of time acupuncture was almost completely abandoned in the early 1960s in many hospitals (evidently because it failed so often), and one authoritative textbook says that fewer than 10,000 operations with it were done in all China during the first eight years it was used for anesthesia. Dr. Bonica doubts it is being used for anesthesia in more than 1 in 10 operations. Moreover, the Chinese statistics would seem to be deliberately misleading in order to build up the value and the status of acupuncture.

Now for the other uses of acupuncture. Dr. Bonica found that no scientific tests of acupuncture had been done, that all reports of its efficacy in helping pain were anecdotal ("this patient was relieved" or "all patients get help" sort of thing). In many health stations and even hospitals no adequate medical records were being kept. And Dr. Bonica could find "no convincing scientific evidence to support the many claims for

. . . acupuncture." But Dr. Bonica has also uncovered some things all interested Americans should be aware of.

THE THREAT AND DANGER OF ACUPUNCTURE

In the same issue of *JAMA* in which Dr. Bonica made his report there was also a series of recent case reports by physicians from the University of Virginia Medical Center in Charlottesville and from the George Washington University Medical Center in Washington, D.C. Although acupuncture is constantly being acclaimed as both effective and safe, neither of these claims is borne out by the facts.

Dr. Bonica, for example, calls attention in *JAMA* to the serious complications that have been reported: death from penetration of the heart by a needle, collapsed lungs, generalized convulsions, the puncturing of the pregnant uterus and of the urinary bladder, paraplegia (paralysis of the lower part of the body and legs), injuries to the liver, spleen and kidneys and a host of other complications.

The team of Virginia and Washington physicians found a middle-aged woman in whom needles placed in the back resulted in breathing difficulties and chest pain; almost a pint of blood had to be drained from her chest, and she suffered for two weeks with a partially collapsed lung and a wound infection. A middle-aged man with asthma stopped using his prescribed steroids and tried acupuncture; on his sixth treatment he suddenly began to fight for breath. Only the availability of a physician and quickly administered oxygen and adrenaline for this acute allergic shock reaction, followed by ambulance transferral to a nearby hospital with an intensive care unit, saved his life.

ACUPUNCTURE FOR YOUR LOW BACK PROBLEMS?

I've been extremely disappointed in the effect of acupuncture on low back dysfunction, and it doesn't seem to do much good for disk disease either. In fact, only when low back problems are divided into two different groups is there evidence of any help from acupuncture.

There are patients who ordinarily do pretty well with a little bed rest, some aspirin, heat or cold, simple back exercises and perhaps some change in their activities. Such patients with simple problems are helped by acupuncture, but they're also helped by a lot of other treatments.

There are also patients who are really incapacitated and ill with their low back problems, who truly can't be active or weight-bearing, can't be on their feet for a long period of time, who have sciatica with changes in their reflexes and muscle weaknesses, who have loss of sensation or paresthesia. There are what we call the real hard neurological pictures where active and aggressive (even surgical) management is necessary. Such patients don't do very well with acupuncture, get little or no help from it.

Dr. Bonica found, in China, claims of good results for chronic back pain—but no hard proof of any long-term success. In fact, one member of his delegation suffered with neck pain from a degenerative disease (spondylolysis) of the cervical vertebrae and tried acupuncture there—without getting any help. Sciatic pain, too, has met only with very uncertain results. Although acupuncture was tried widely for arthritis, the Chinese could provide no scientific proof of success.

At the June, 1973, Annual Scientific Session of the Arthritis Foundation, a University of California medical team reported on their study of the effect of acupuncture on rheumatoid arthritis. There was no improvement in the disease itself, although the needles did seem to help the pain, as did sham acupuncture (putting the needles in the wrong places, or only superficially, not twirling them). The California team concluded: " . . . a placebo effect contributed at least partially to the observed analgesia."

In short, this Stone Age treatment at this point seems to offer nothing that can't be equaled or bettered in other ways, and certainly there is no scientific proof that it really helps low back problems, that it does any more than any one of a flock of other treatments from aspirin to sugar pills. Moreover, for your own protection you should recognize that acupuncture is neither completely safe nor totally harmless. It will, of course, be interesting to see what happens as this treatment loses its newness, for this alone traditionally has made remedies work, has resulted in cures which time and familiarity soon cause to lose their power.

Alpha: Fact or Fiction?

From what one reads or hears or sees in the varied news media one might think that everybody's "into alpha" these days—and without really knowing what alpha actually is. Back in 1929 a Bavarian director of the psychiatric clinic at Jena, Germany—Dr. Hans Berger—built the first electroencephalogram (EEG in medical shorthand), an electronic device which picks up electrical changes in the brain. The EEG amplifies an electrical current more than a million times and so is able to detect and record even the tiny amounts of electricity—some one ten-thousandth of a volt—which the brain continuously generates.

Berger named the different types of brain waves he found in the order he discovered them, using the Greek alphabet—alpha, beta, theta and delta. These are rhythmically oscillating waves put out by the brain at either 8 to 12 waves per second (alpha), 13 to 25 (beta) and so on. Those known as delta waves may arise from areas of localized damage (scar tissue or a brain tumor, for example).

The EEG has become a vital medical tool, revealing many problems such as epilepsy, tumors or other brain conditions. It has also been used in a new approach—biofeedback. This method concerns itself with detecting any biological changes (muscle contraction, alpha brain waves, heart rate) and then feeding information about these changes (increased alpha waves, decreased muscle contraction, slower or faster heart rate) back by any one of a variety of means—a light or a sound tone or just a squiggle along a strip of paper (such as an electrocardiograph makes). Just the awareness of one's own bodily changes has produced changes and claims of many things accomplished—control of migraine and epilepsy and blood pressure, of blood supply to a hand and much more.

British doctors of the last century brought back from India reports of yogis who stopped their heart from beating, at will, were even buried underground and dug up alive. These were all discounted in the West, although Dr. Paul Dudley White proved it in 1917 while only a young resident at Massachusetts General Hospital. A medical student said he could speed up his heart, so young Dr. White dragged him off to his laboratory and attached the student to an early electrocardiograph and told him to demonstrate.

As magnificent old Dr. White recalled before his recent death: "One second later his heart began to accelerate, and he reached a rate of 140 to 150 [normally it's about 70] within a few seconds by willpower. His pupils dilated. His blood pressure went up." Young Dr. White reported it—and also discovered that the chief of surgery was able to do it too, even though he hadn't done so in seventeen years. Dr. White was chagrined: "It seems so queer I didn't realize the importance of this fifty years ago."

In the late 1960s Rockefeller University's Dr. Neal Miller and his associates taught rats to lower their heart rates from 350 beats a minute to a mere 230, to make one ear blush and the other pale, to increase and decrease blood pressure, intestinal contractions, urine excretion and other bodily functions. And at the Menninger Foundation, an Indian yogi was able recently to jump his heart beat from 70 to 300 and make two spots only a couple of inches apart on his palm warm and cool so that there was a 10° F differential. Ordinary Americans also have proved able to warm their hands as much as 10° and so control their migraine attacks when they learned to warm their hands by means of biofeedback (a temperature-sensing device connected to their hands told them when they were succeeding). And at Denver's University of Colorado, other Americans have learned with biofeedback to relax their head muscles and end their tension headaches.

Still others have learned to control spasms of the hand arteries (Raynaud's disease) at Massachusetts General Hospital. Reports tell of research endeavors (still unproved) to lower blood pressure (from 140 to 70 in one woman), speed or slow heart rate and eliminate that organ's irregularities.

BIOFEEDBACK, ALPHA AND LOW BACK PROBLEMS

Of potential significance to our special interest is the report that this training restores muscle function in people who have suffered paralysis of half their bodies or slight paralysis of the lower limbs. However, we certainly cannot at this time consider biofeedback as a part of our routine medical armamentarium.

BIOFEEDBACK—FROM THE OTHER SIDE

In all the flood of exciting reports of the miracles of biofeedback, the strong popular movement of being "into alpha," only now has come a voice from the other side, a coldly scientific appraisal and assessment of this new field. In the May, 1974, *Archives of General Psychiatry* is an article by a team headed by Dr. Edward B. Blanchard. In this critical scientific review of biofeedback training the team came to the conclusion that there are actually only very limited areas in which there is acceptable and strong support for the efficacy of this new medical tool.

Close to proved is the work in muscle training such as tension headaches and in muscle retraining which involves paralysis. These are the very areas which may prove of help in low back problems, where muscle problems such as lumbosacral strains and many vague backaches owing to tension are involved. The possibilities look exciting, too, in paralysis, for this does happen when there are injuries to the spinal cord or the cauda equina or the spinal nerve roots. In many of the other uses to which biofeedback has been put and which we have mentioned there is often suggestive but nowhere any conclusive evidence.

Chiropractic and Manipulation—and Your Aching Back

Chiropractic was founded by Daniel David Palmer in 1895 and is based on the supposed principle that the cause of disease can be found and corrected with the hands because illness is due to an abnormal functioning of the nervous system—along with almost metaphysical vague discussions of matter movement and mental energy. Therapy is a matter—according to chiropractors—of restoring normal function to to the nervous system by manipulation of the body, especially the spinal column.

The organized medical profession has long attacked chiropractic as unscientific cultism which should be discarded and ignored, while the chiropractors have accused the physicians of being financially motivated bigots. Perhaps the closest thing to an unbiased investigation was made by the U.S. Department of Health, Education, and Welfare in 1968, when in a report to Congress it stated: "Chiropractic theory and practice are not based upon the body of basic knowledge related to health disease, and health care that has been widely accepted by the scientific community. Moreover, irrespective of its theory, the scope and quality of chiropractic education do not prepare the practitioner to make an adequate diagnosis and provide appropriate treatment. . . ."

In another federal report in 1967 the number of practicing chiropractors in the United States was put at between 14,000 and 35,000, and the numbers of patients they treated at as high as 3,000,000 a year. One can only speculate that with this many patients these practitioners must be giving their patients something, but what need they fill is something else again. For there are many psychosomatic disorders, many emotional problems, which seek satisfaction in a variety of forms of unscientific cultism, in bizarre forms of healing or diets or whatever—or in the sugar pills the wise physician has always used effectively and safely.

CHIROPRACTIC AND MANIPULATION: THE GOOD AND THE BAD

Chiropractic is no panacea, can even certainly be treacherous in effect (used on a patient whose underlying problem is cancer, it can delay proper care and conceivably cost the patient his life), but the value of its manipulation can be very real, although limited.

Only recently a pair of neurologists at the University of California at San Francisco reported on a dozen instances of stroke either induced or related to chiropractic treatment. Most patients were under the age of forty, and exactly how this happens isn't understood. Two patients the California neurologists described might be of value as a warning. A fifty-two-year-old woman with neck pain developed dizziness, nausea and blurred vision during the treatment, followed by weakness and numbness on the left side. After nearly a half year of medical therapy, strength and coordination were only partially regained.

And a thirty-five-year-old former serviceman suffered similar symptoms after a chiropractic adjustment for a stiff, aching neck. He lost consciousness during the first manipulation, but a second one was still administered, and now he suffered blurred vision, vomiting, inability to sit or stand and difficulty with his memory. After a year of neurological treatment, he was still severely handicapped.

Manipulation, however, is one of the oldest forms of therapy, having been used by Hippocrates, and its origins are lost in history. During the eighteenth and nineteenth centuries the bonesetters in England were well known for this form of treatment and kept their special methods within families, passing the secrets down from generation to generation. In fact, Mrs. Sally Mapp, a noted English bonesetter, was so successful in eighteenth-century London that she was paid by the town of Epsom to live there and drove into London twice a week in a magnificent coach-and-four, with gorgeously liveried servants.

While there have been instances where manipulation of the low back has caused severe flare-ups, there has been an awakening of medical interest in recent years, especially among those active in the treatment of low back dysfunction. It is effective under certain circumstances. Its help may arise from the stretching of muscles and tendons already short-ened and contracted from spasm and may be related to some alteration in the lumbar facet joints. Perhaps the fibrous tis-sue around these joints becomes contracted and even devel-ops adhesions from prolonged immobility of the lower back. However, there is no basis to claims that manipulation pro-duces an "adjustment" or realignment of the subluxated, or partially dislocated, vertebrae.

Many patients with chronic intermittent low back pain will routinely seek manipulative therapy when their pain be-comes acute, and a sizable number of them derive symp-tomatic relief from this treatment. Sometimes the results will be striking, and a person who is barely able to hobble into the office because of his acute pain will stride out comfortably al-most immediately after a manipulative session.

The clicking or cracking sounds during manipulation oc-cur in almost nine out of ten of those who receive manipula-tion on a regular basis, but in less than one out of four of those who've never had it before. The exact cause of the clicking has never been clearly explained to my satisfaction, but it might be produced by a vacuum phenomenon at the facet joints similar to the pop which occurs when some peo-ple crack their knuckles.

Before one even considers this treatment, a complete eval-uation and examination, including low back spinal X rays, should be done. A number of disorders are distinct contrain-dications, such as tumors, vertebral fractures, dislocations and the like. No properly performed manipulation should cause discomfort to the normal patient, and the session shouldn't be particularly painful even for low back sufferers.

The maneuvers used are varied and may be a matter of the physician's placing his hands on the patient's back and making a series of short, rapid thrusts, using the heels of his hands. Or the legs may be raised or rotated, or the body rotated. If you decide to undergo this therapy, you should have definite improvement of your symptoms after the first session. If there's no relief, the condition will not respond to this treatment, and there is no use in a repeat.

Chapter 18

HOME REMEDIES FOR YOUR LOW BACK DISCOMFORTS:
The Miracle Drug for Your Pain, Hot and Cold, Massage—and When to Call the Doctor

YOUR MEDICINE cabinet at home contains a whole variety of things for help in the minor everyday medical problems, and this chapter is meant to do the same for your low back. Here are the home remedies, all the way from a true miracle drug that's almost always available to tricks in handling hot and cold, which to apply and when. But the first subject, of course, is when to call for help.

When Should You Call Your Doctor for Your Low Back?

This is always a tricky question and not the easiest thing in the world to know, even for your doctor. First, we all usually know when *not* to call the doctor. If you get a backache after you've played tennis for the first time in the year, if you've worked too long in the garden or just finished the spring housecleaning, and after an aspirin or two, a hot tub or a heating pad, it all begins to feel better, if the pain is mainly stiffness and leaves you decreasingly uncomfortable for only a day or two before it's gone, surely you don't need a doctor. In fact, if you ran in to see him every time this sort of thing happened, he would only be annoyed, and with today's medical fees you probably couldn't afford it anyhow.

But how about those pains which come on without any cause you can find? Here a lot depends on two factors: the severity and the length of time it lasts. The all-out severe kind decides for itself. If you can't straighten up after bending over, if you have to be lifted up to be moved, if the pain is unbearable, there will be no question in your mind; you'll know you have to call for help.

But you might well put the dividing line between the backaches for which you call the doctor and those for which you don't at the point where pain interferes with your daily living activities. If you can't carry out your job or care for your children, if you can't go about your ordinary daily activities, obviously you need medical help.

But what of the pain that's not incapacitating? This is where you need some guidelines, when you want to know what to do. The pain is there, you can get around and do your work, but it hurts. Let's say you've never had this particular pain before, for some people are plagued with backaches, have had them diagnosed and know they're only chronic unimportant nuisances. Then the test is whether it appeared, say, on a Monday, and when you got up on Tuesday, it was still there and as bad or worse. If you've done nothing to set if off (say, strain your back), you might well begin to wonder about seeing your doctor—and I would suggest you do see him either on Tuesday or certainly on Wednesday if the pain is still there.On the other hand, if it's a strain and you know it, and it yields to simple home care and doesn't come back, why, you're home free and can forget it.

In short, when there's any change in your normal health pattern—and the amount or severity of the pain isn't the final arbiter except when it's overwhelming—it's time to think about medical help unless it's a passing thing, a pain of a few moments, for example. If the change lasts into a second day, it's certainly time to wonder about what's going on and take some action, say a call for medical advice or an actual visit to your physician.

The same is true if the pain, however mild, keeps recurring even if it doesn't last. Prompt medical help can prevent many serious complications, can abort a variety of health problems or catch other disorders in time to prevent major trouble. Actually this sort of defensive thinking is good for almost any health problem. *When in doubt, call your doctor.* And remember, pain isn't the only warning signal.

NONPAINFUL WARNING SIGNALS IN BACK AND LEGS

Where low back problems occur, pain is only one of many warning signals—and often not the most serious. If you think back for a moment to the chapter on disk problems, you will recall some of the effects that nerve root pressure or pressure on the cauda equina or the spinal cord itself can produce. In fact, these "neurological" symptoms are very often far more serious than many of the back pains which may only be a sign of passing minor muscular strains.

Should you notice any numbness or loss of sensation in the low back, the buttocks or legs or feet—such an occurrence most certainly warrants prompt medical attention. No one need tell you that if there is any paralysis, you should call a doctor. But sometimes this takes the form of minor muscular weaknesses to begin with—a tripping over little things such as curbs or rocks or the edge of rugs; some difficulty in climbing stairs when there is a feeling of a leg giving out from under you unexpectedly.

Another warning signal is paresthesia—the strange sensations which may appear in low back, buttocks, legs or feet. These may be a sensation of insects crawling over the skin, itching or tickling, pricking or tingling, burning or cold or pins and needles. In short, any unusual or unnatural sensation is a cause for concern and a doctor.

A very serious symptom is any difficulty with bowel or bladder control, and this should send you posthaste to your doctor. Difficulty in voiding calls for a prompt medical opinion, and even a sudden onset of constipation may be the first indication of muscle involvement. When there is serious nerve involvement through the pressure of herniated disks or tumors there may be impairment of the muscles guarding the bladder and rectal portals so that voiding becomes affected.

You may even notice an atrophy or shrinkage of the muscles in thigh or calf of one leg, although this will likely be too slight for you to notice. A tape measure will quickly confirm any marked atrophy simply by comparing the size of the two legs. Again—*if there is any question, see a doctor.* But what of home care?

Should You Use Hot or Cold?

The best answer to whether to use hot or cold for that aching back which doesn't need a doctor—the minor overuse or strain—is the story of the man for whose backache his doctor prescribed heat. Four weeks went by without relief. Hobbling up to his club's bar, he complained of his lack of relief to his favorite bartender, who promptly advised the use of cold. In desperation the executive went home and tried ice on his back. The next day he was fine, and there was no more trouble. Angry that his doctor hadn't advised him to use cold during his miserable month, he reproached his physician with the nonprofessional advice that worked so well. His doctor looked up at him and replied, "That's funny. My bartender always advises heat."

I think any physician who limits his advice to either heat or cold is failing to recognize that neither one always works— and we really don't know why. When one doesn't work, I try the other; there is no way to tell in advance which is going to work.

Cold is one of the most ancient means of controlling pain, and surely prehistoric man knew that putting an aching arm or leg in a cold stream relieved the pain. Gradually it became obvious that even surgery could be performed by numbing the limb with cold.

Dominique Larrey, Napoleon's surgeon in chief, used ice to produce refrigeration anesthesia for amputations during the Russian campaign, and this is still being used for this type of surgery and has much to recommend it. Refrigeration was also introduced for local anesthesia as a result of Sir Benjamin W. Richardson (an English physician of the mid-nineteenth century) having some cologne placed on his forehead and blown on. Noticing it made the skin numb, he soon tried ether for evaporating on a patient's skin and obtained local anesthesia for simple procedures. Today ethyl chloride is widely used by both doctor and dentist for this same purpose.

The use of cold for muscle aches and pains was first introduced to modern medicine from its use in professional athletics, where managers are interested not in curing but in getting the athlete back into action as soon as possible. For minor injuries in a game they either spray the area with ethyl chloride or some other more effective modern agent or simply rub the injury with an ice lollipop (we'll discuss this in just a moment). But trainers and team doctors noticed that not only was the athlete able to get back into the game, but the injury felt much better later on. As a result, a host of doctors interested in muscular problems of the low back suddenly began using cold for these dysfunctions.

HOW TO APPLY HEAT AND COLD

You can make your own ice lollipops by putting a wooden stick (we use ordinary tongue depressors) in a can filled with water and freezing it. Running warm water over the can will allow you to slip it off and free the ice lollipop for use. Then run the ice back and forth over the area that's bothering you. Of course, you can also use a simple ice bag or ice wrapped in a plastic cap or even a towel. Once the part or area has become numb, keep the ice on for *no more* than another five seconds.

Refrigerant sprays too are helpful but should *be used only with your doctor's advice*, since he can show you how to do it safely without hurting yourself. Many of these are explosive, can produce skin burns if misused and are dangerous when inhaled. Ethyl chloride is an anesthetic and must be handled with considerable care.

Most convenient and simplest to use are the new gels which can be frozen and reused repeatedly. Encased in a plastic container, they are simple to use and effective—but should be applied for *only five seconds after* the skin becomes numb. They can then be stored away.

Heat, too, is available in a whole slew of forms today, from the simplest home applications to the Space Age techniques of the doctor's office. The use of heat too goes back to prehistoric people, who must early have noticed how good the sun felt on aches and bruises. The ancient Egyptians and Greeks and other primitive peoples all utilized heat in their medical practices.

You can apply it in the most simple and ancient way by soaking in a hot tub for half an hour or so. If the water seems cool after a while, just swish it around since your body will take the heat out of the water next to it. Another way of applying moist heat is a turkish towel soaked in hot water—*with care* because this can burn you if it's too hot, as can the mud type of packs that are now available to be *used with care* for a half hour or so to avoid burns.

Whether moist or dry heat is preferable is another unresolved question. Moist heat is generally regarded as preferable, but the answer depends on which works best in any particular instance. Dry heat can consist of soaking in the sun or of using the new heat-retaining gels which can be reused—both to be applied *with care*. And there is the electric heating pad which is safest when wrapped in a dry turkish towel and used *with care* and placed on, *not under*, the body to avoid burns. Use of heat or infrared lamp carries all the same precautions and is best applied with a turkish towel on your body. Be very careful that you *do not fall asleep while applying heat.*

Your doctor may utilize special types of infrared lamps. The shortwave diathermy machine sets the molecules in your body moving so that heat is produced deep in the tissues.

The newest and deepest form of heat treatment is the ultrasound which utilizes sound waves beyond the range of human hearing. These penetrate deep into tissues and joints but must be handled skillfully to avoid any damage. Even microwave diathermy is available, but its value has been questioned; it is intermediate between shortwave and ultrasound in the depth to which it penetrates.

Whether deep heat is any better than the hot tub or the heating pad is still questionable. In most instances the heat or cold is there to get you over a particular incident, not to cure the problem. If a difficulty recurs, more is needed than heat or cold therapy. If, when the treatment is over, the pain or spasm comes back without any real improvement time after time, you need more than this therapy, and proper, even specialized, medical care is called for.

Massage

The use of massage also goes back before recorded history. And this, too, has its role in the conservative treatment of low back dysfunctions. Spasms of the low back muscles can often be relaxed by a gently performed, deep-kneading type of massage. This helps because it increases the blood flow, relaxes the muscles and improves the spasm.

Besides this deep-kneading type of massage, there is the simple stroking or gentle rubbing which anyone in the family can do, and this too often helps. For one thing just the simple laying on of hands is relaxing to many people and is often the basis of much healing, of the help that a nurse or doctor provides a patient simply by patting or holding a hand or an arm. How much of this psychological help is involved in massaging really isn't known.

Another form of massage is called skin rolling. This is effective for areas where there is soreness or aching and where the doctor hasn't found anything wrong beyond some muscle spasms. A skin fold is lifted up and then rolled along the body surface. This takes a bit of doing and some practice—and may be acutely painful if it's done right over the aching area. But after such a treatment the sufferer often finds considerable improvement in both symptoms and discomfort.

Finally, the ice lollipop can be used effectively for massaging the painful area. There are quite a number of other massage techniques, but these are for the skilled physiotherapist, who has a wide range of such methods at his command.

Miracle Drug and Pain-killer: Cure-all and Killer

It was used back in the Stone Age and by Hippocrates and the North American Indians; it was even in the medical kits of our astronauts on their voyages to the moon. It's not much better understood now than it was in the Stone Age, even though it's now manufactured by the hundreds of billions of tablets. One of the safest of drugs, it's also one of the leading killers of little children. More than any other single drug, it can be truly termed a miracle drug, and it's the chief weapon against arthritis and more valuable than any other in low back problems.

This amazing drug is aspirin. It's probably the most powerful analgesic pound for pound when taken by mouth. Only recently it has been found more effective against the pain of abdominal cancer than the routinely used oral narcotic codeine. It's a powerful anti-inflammatory drug which is still the mainstay of antiarthritic therapy. All of which resulted in 1970 in 17,500 *tons* of aspirin being consumed—225 tablets for every American man, woman, and child, 60,000,000 to 75,000,000 tablets each and every day.

Aspirin—acetylsalicylic acid, chemically—is a member of a family called the salicylates. These are found widely in nature in trees (the willow in particular), in shrubs and various fruits and have been used since the Stone Age. In the form of willow leaves and bark and roots, Hippocrates advised it for childbirth, Roman soldiers used it for fevers, ancient

Greeks and medieval people all utilized the analgesic qualities of these fabulous chemicals.

More than any other drug known to man, aspirin can be regarded as the universal analgesic, but there are two things you should know about this miracle drug: its dangers and the ways to take and to buy it.

THE DANGERS OF ASPIRIN

Aspirin is probably the safest of all drugs when you stop to consider the enormous amounts consumed and the few reactions. But it can be dangerous, for it does kill a hundred or so children every year, along with an uncounted number of adolescents and adults. Its chief danger with children is the fact that it is so safe that adults forget that large amounts do poison children, who will bolt down anything they can get their hands on—particularly if it's candy-coated.

More than any other drug, aspirin is a matter of one man's meat being another man's poison; as few as 3 aspirin have killed some adults, while others have survived as many as 430 tablets. While millions take it safely, 2 persons in every 1,000 are hypersensitive and have a violent and sometimes fatal reaction without warning and even after having taken it earlier without problems. About 5 percent of people will get heartburn from just a single tablet, while some experts feel that even one tablet causes loss of blood from the gastrointestinal tract. Serious loss of hearing has resulted from as few as 3 tablets. Yet many arthritics who are not sensitive to the drug can take as many as 20 tablets a day for decades without trouble.

Since it affects blood clotting, aspirin is dangerous for those with stomach ulcers, those taking blood thinners or other drugs—and for asthmatics in particular. If you are taking *any* drug, you should check with your doctor before taking even a single aspirin. In fact, *to be safe,* you should really *check with your doctor before you take that first aspirin.*

WHAT TO BUY IN ASPIRIN AND HOW TO TAKE IT

All aspirin is the same—as long as it's labeled USP (United States Pharmacopoeia) and has the same strength (for adults usually 5 grains or 300 milligrams). In short, the cheaper the brand, the better the buy as long as it fulfills these requirements. However, aspirin is also available in forms which can be more effective or which can avoid stomach irritation. Your doctor will be the one to decide this. For occasional home use you're better off with straight aspirin, and you can take it either after a meal or with some antacid to avoid the heartburn you hear some people complain of.

RUBBING IT IN

A number of other salicylates—cousins of aspirin—are also available for direct application. Oil of wintergreen (methyl salicylate) is an effective analgesic rub on the painful low back area.

Stocking Your Low Back Medicine Cabinet

For the help you want for those occasional minor low back problems, you can stock your medicine cabinet with a few simple safe items. Aspirin (USP 5-grain tablets for adults) is the big gun here—and some antacid to take with it. There are gels which can be frozen for cold applications and some tongue depressors, along with a can or two for making ice lollipops. And there are the heat-retaining gels or mud type of packs. In some convenient spot you might also want to keep an electric heating pad, and you might even want an infrared lamp.

Chapter 19

THE EXERCISES FOR YOUR LOW BACK:
How to Keep Away from the Doctor

THE VERY word "exercise" is often misleading to patient and physician alike. All too often the picture that arises in the mind is one of gymnastics, of strenuous athletics with a Charles Atlas the end result. But while there is certainly no objection to your developing a muscular physique, becoming an athlete or a gymnast, this really has nothing whatsoever to do with our specific objectives.

In fact, many low back sufferers are actually trim, are often splendid tennis players or golfers who certainly don't need any further physical or muscular development. And all you need do is follow the sports pages in your daily newspaper to learn of the professional athletes in many contact sports who are plagued by back problems.

Low back dysfunction isn't necessarily a matter of not doing sufficient exercises or physical work but one of not giving certain muscles enough activity—or the right kinds—to keep them in proper tone and condition. It's also a matter of improper posture. The vast majority of people who show improper posture usually have an increased lumbar lordosis (swayback or saddleback). Because of this, many of the low back exercise programs are designed to flatten out or at least to reduce this lordosis, essentially to flatten the low back.

The Secret of the Exercises

The success of exercises depends on two factors: the pa-

223

tient and the doctor. The patient must be prepared to carry out his exercises day in and day out, and here is the problem, for it's hard to get people to continue this on a lifetime basis. Yet on this depends your hope—if you are one of those with faulty posture or low back muscles in poor condition—for a pain-free life so far as your low back is concerned.

All too often a standard set of back exercises is handed to sufferers with little or no instruction, and they are left to find their own way, to plan a regimen for their own special problems all by themselves. The result is not going to be successful, for the management of any low back problem demands personal individual attention—whether it be the determination of the amount and kind of rest (total bed rest, eight hours' sleep, afternoon nap and the like), decisions about wearing a low back support (the kind and the times), medication to be used (aspirin or muscle relaxants or whatever) and so on.

There are four special areas of individual concern in planning any low back exercise program. First there is the specific postural impairment of the particular sufferer. Secondly, there is the need for a pre-exercise evaluation to determine the strength and flexibility of the chief muscle groups involved. Thirdly, there is the matter of allowing for the special effects of the various exercises on the chief muscle groups. Fourthly, there is the degree of muscle strength and flexibility needed for each exercise and the determination of whether the patient is up to this demand.

A Warning About Low Back Exercises

It is essential that you *check with your doctor before attempting any exercise; you must be sure that the exercise will help you, that the exercise is not wrong or harmful for you.* Only the doctor who knows your general health and the condition of your low back as well can decide this.

You must be sure to *do these every single day.* The on-again, off-again pattern isn't going to accomplish anything except waste your time and leave you with the old backache and the feeling that the exercises aren't doing any good.

When Do You Start Back Exercises and Where Do You Do Them?

Again, ask your doctor. But in general, this program of low back exercises is started as soon as pain relief has been achieved with bed rest and other conservative measures. It may be begun with several sessions of massage and diathermy for both abdominal and low back muscles, to prepare the way for the exercises, which can at first be done on a flattened bed. Once your condition permits it, a firmer surface—a mat- or rug-covered floor—is preferable because it allows easier maneuverability and greater awareness of points of body contact.

Testing Your Muscles

The first step the doctor will take before prescribing exercises will be to evaluate both the strength and the flexibility of the low back muscles by means of tests.

Abdominal strength: Stretched out flat on your back with your hands clasped behind your neck, you keep your knees straight and lift your feet twelve inches off the floor or other hard flat surface. If you can keep this position for ten seconds, you have normal lower abdominal muscle strength.

Now your doctor or anyone else holds your feet against the floor while you're stretched out flat on your back. If you can now do a sit-up—lift your trunk from the floor to a straight-up or 90-degree sitting position—you have normal upper abdominal muscle strength.

The degree to which you fail fully to perform this and the next tests indicates the extent to which your muscles are deficient: Lift your legs six inches, and you have 50 percent of normal lower abdominal strength. The aim in prescribing exercises is to concentrate on restoring your muscle weaknesses or lack of elasticity, and the tests provide a measurement to tell the extent of your deficiencies and then measure their restoration to normal.

Lumbar strength: While stretched out flat on your stomach with a pillow under your abdomen and your legs held against the floor, you have to lift your chest off the surface on which you're lying. If you can maintain this position for ten seconds, you have normal upper back muscle strength.

Again flat on your stomach with the pillow under your abdomen, your chest is held against the floor by hands pressing down on your shoulders. Now you have to lift your legs off the surface. If you can hold your legs up this way for ten seconds, you have normal lower back muscle strength.

Lumbar and hamstring elasticity (the hamstring is the pair of tendons on the inside hollow of your knee): Stand up straight with your bare or stockinged feet together, keep your knees straight and bend forward, trying to touch the floor with your fingertips. If you can touch the floor, you have normal lumbar muscle and hamstring elasticity, but if you can't, measure the distance from your fingertips to the floor. Take twenty-four inches as the starting point. If you miss the floor by eighteen inches, it means you have a 75 percent deficiency in elasticity, twelve inches short means a 50 percent deficiency and so on.

This test is important in that long-standing muscle tension produces a lack of mechanical elasticity or a relative muscle contracture which also makes the muscle less flexible. Some experts feel that tension and spasticity affecting the low back muscle makes this area more vulnerable to mechanical trauma and leads to recurrent lumbosacral strain.

How to Set Up Your Exercise Program

Never do either the muscle strength tests or the exercises during a period of acute pain. Only after the pain is gone should you establish your exercise program.

To accomplish any satisfactory results, you must develop

regularity in performing your low back exercises twice a day without fail. It's particularly important that even on days which involve considerable emotional stress or increased amounts of work, time should be set aside for these exercises. In fact, it is probably during these very times of heightened stress or work that the exercises will prove most helpful.

Remember: An erratic exercise program is virtually worthless.

How to Relax Before Your Exercises: Important!

All low back exercise programs should include relaxation and limbering-up exercises before you get down to your low back because otherwise you'll be working against tense muscles which will prevent any effective help in either developing strength or improving elasticity. If you don't relax first, you'll be wasting almost all the effort and time you put into your exercises, and if you don't first limber up your muscles, you may strain the muscles instead of helping them.

1. While lying on the floor, raise your arms slowly over your head as you inhale deeply. Then exhale as you allow your arms to return slowly to the floor. Do this ten times, and with each exhalation allow your arms and legs, head and shoulders to rest limply on the floor, letting your entire body go soft and limp.

2. Breathe deeply, and with each slow inhalation, bring your legs and feet tightly together, arms tightly at your side. Make tight fists; tighten all the muscles of your entire body, including those of your buttocks. Then with each exhalation relax as completely as possible, allowing your arms and legs to "drift away" from your body, closing your eyes and allowing even your jaw to sag. Repeat ten times.

This alternation of muscle contraction with relaxation is a helpful trick to increase the relaxation. By directing your attention to the difference between muscle tension and muscle relaxation, you can accentuate the relaxation. Done properly, each succeeding relaxation is a bit more profound, produces greater total physical and mental relaxation. When this has all been completed, you are ready to start your low back exercises.

The Pelvic Tuck or Uptilt

The most essential of all the corrective low back exercises is some variation of the pelvic "tuck or uptilt," for this accustoms the muscles to eliminate or at least to reduce the lumbar lordosis. This is a simple exercise which can begin as soon as the acute attack of low back pain or muscle spasm has eased, even while the patient is still in bed. Later it is performed on the floor.

You must avoid the common error of lifting the low back along with the buttocks and thus curving instead of flattening the lumbar spine. Depending on your response and your doctor's advice, the bend of the hip and knees is reduced until both are out flat, which increases the flattening of the spine. After two weeks or more of this advanced pelvic tuck, the exercise should be practiced while standing upright against a wall.

These are a pair of exercises designed to stretch the muscles which flex or bend your hip.

Corrective Low Back Exercises

These exercises are graded into three phases which provide steadily increasing work to improve the condition of your low back:

Phase 1: These are the exercises prescribed for those patients who have only recently recovered from a bout of low back pain. They should be performed twice a day for one month. If after this time there is no difficulty with carrying out these exercises, you may then go on to the next set.

Phase 2: These exercises are done after doing a set of Phase 1 exercises which act as preliminaries to limber you up. This is also done twice a day for four months. If everything goes well with these, you will be ready for the final Phase 3.

FINNESON CORRECTIVE LOW BACK EXERCISE PROGRAM
PELVIC UPTILT

1. Lie flat on back with knees bent and feet flat on floor.
2. Flatten entire spine against floor.
3. Keeping back flat on floor, raise buttocks up (pelvic uptilt) by contracting stomach and buttock muscles.
4. Repeat ten times.

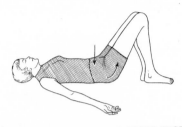

ILIOPSOAS STRETCHING EXERCISES

1. Lie flat on back with both legs extended.
2. Pull right knee up to chest, keeping left leg extended.
3. Press back firmly against floor.
4. Straighten right leg, and pull left knee up to chest.
5. Repeat five times with each leg.

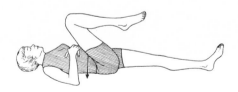

1. Kneel on right knee.
2. Place left leg in front of you with foot flat on floor.
3. Place hands on floor on either side of left leg for balance.
4. Extend right leg behind you.
5. Position now is similar to that of a racing start.
6. Rock back and forth between right and left leg ten times.
7. Repeat with right leg forward ten times.

Regular Exercises and Isometrics: Advantages and Draw-backs

FINNESON CORRECTIVE LOW BACK EXERCISE PROGRAM
PHASE 1 EXERCISES

1. a. Lie flat on back on floor.
    b. Bend knees as much as possible.
    c. Slowly allow them to return to start position limp and relaxed.
    d. Repeat five times.

2. a. Lie flat on back with knees bent.
    b. Bring both knees up to chest, and clasp tightly with hands.
    c. Hold position for count of ten.
    d. Return to starting position.
    e. Repeat three times.

3. a. Lie flat on back with legs extended.
    b. Clasp hands behind head.
    c. Raise right knee up toward chest as far as possible.
    d. Hold for count of ten.
    e. Return to start position.
    f. Repeat with left leg.
    g. Repeat five times with each leg.

4. a. Lie flat on back with arms above head and knees bent.
    b. Flatten back against floor, and contract stomach muscles.
    c. Hold for count of ten.
    d. Repeat five times.

5. a. Sit in a chair with hands at your side.
    b. Drop head down between knees.
    c. Allow hands to rest on floor.
    d. Hold position for count of three.
    e. Return to sitting position.
    f. Repeat five times.

FINNESON CORRECTIVE LOW BACK EXERCISE PROGRAM
PHASE 2 EXERCISES

Continue to do relaxation exercises, pelvic uptilt, hip flexion and all Phase 1 exercises before starting on these. Do pelvic uptilt exercise with legs extended instead of knees bent.

1.   a. Lie flat on back with knees bent and feet flat on floor.
       b. Rotate hips and legs to right side, keeping feet flat on floor.
       c. Then return to straight position.
       d. Rotate to opposite side.
       e. Repeat five times each side.

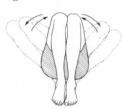

2.   a. Lie flat on back with legs extended.
       b. Raise feet twelve inches off floor and hold for count of ten.
       c. Slowly lower feet to floor.
       d. Repeat five times.

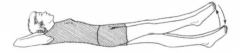

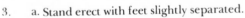

3.   a. Stand erect with feet slightly separated.
       b. Hold onto chair or table for balance.
       c. Sit down.
       d. Straighten up.
       e. Repeat five times (do not use table to
          pull yourself up—just to maintain balance).

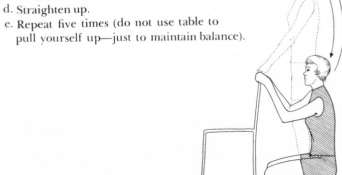

4.   a. Lie flat on back with legs extended.
      b. Raise right leg as far as possible without bending knee.
      c. Lower slowly to floor.
      d. Repeat with left leg.
      e. Repeat five times with each leg.

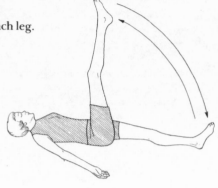

5.   a. Lie flat on back with legs extended.
      b. Bend right.knee, and place right foot against left knee.
      c. Keeping sole of foot touching knee, rotate right knee to right (aim
         is to get knee as close to floor as possible).
      d. Return right knee to upright position.
      e. Then rotate knee toward left side as far as possible.
      f. Return to start position.
      g. Repeat with left foot against right knee.
      h. Alternate sides until exercise is done five times with each leg.

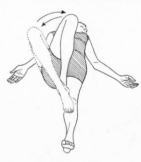

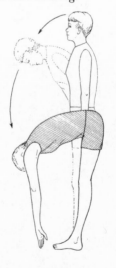

6.   a. Stand erect with legs slightly separated.
      b. Bend head, neck and finally body forward from the hips.
      c. Keep knees straight, and try to touch the floor with your finger-
         tips.
      d. Repeat five times.

Phase 3: These are the most strenuous exercises and are done to maintain the low back and abdominal musculature in the healthy condition they should now be in. Here you lie on your back with your hands clasped behind your head, your feet tucked under a heavy object (say, a sofa or chair). Now do a sit-up until your body is up at a 90-degree angle to your legs, and then slowly lower yourself to a lying position. Repeat this ten times. The rest of Phase 3 is really a matter of maintaining your low back health, and this your doctor can decide. Perhaps he will advise walking or bicycling or jogging or swimming on a regular basis and set the amount and pattern for your age and condition—and your likes or dislikes.

A lot of the exercises we have been describing will—at the same time that they strengthen abdominal and back muscles—put a strain on the low back structures. It has been shown by actually measuring the pressure in the nucleus pulposus of the spinal disks that in doing sit-ups, for example, you actually put the spinal disks under a good deal of pressure. If one assumes that some of the low back problems with a certain degree of lumbar disk dysfunction have some disk weakness or bulge in addition to weak muscles, then in strengthening these muscles by regular exercises such as sit-ups, you may be further weakening the disks and may conceivably cause problems.

Isometric exercises, on the other hand, don't put any more stress on the disk than does standing or sitting, so you run less risk of causing any intrinsic damage to the disk. Although isometric exercises are just as good for building up the abdominal muscle tone and strength as are the regular exercises, you also help all the trunk muscles. If you try tightening up your abdominal muscles, you will feel how all the other trunk muscles tighten up as well, so you get general help for all your torso musculature.

In a similar fashion, if you tuck up your pelvis isometrically you also straighten out the lumbar lordosis. You can do this simply by tightening up your abdominal muscles while you sit on your chair reading this. Isometric exercises, however, also have their shortcomings, for they fail to produce the suppleness and elasticity that the regular exercises will produce in the muscles, ligaments and tendons of the entire torso.

Isometric exercises when done regularly will certainly add support to your back. But while they will reduce the need for some of the other exercises, they do not displace them. Moreover, you have to do more of the isometrics. Many patients feel they're not accomplishing anything with isometrics and so are likely to get careless with them. Many patients also consider them boring and fail to perform them regularly.

The Isometric Exercises

These have to be done on a regular basis, too, if they are to accomplish anything. More of these are needed than the regular exercises to gain the same amount of muscle strengthening and tone improvement. Isometrics should be done for fifteen minutes two or three times a day. Tighten the stomach muscles (even tuck up your pelvis), and hold them this way for a second or two at a time; then let go.

One trick is to carry out this exercise during driving. Every time you stop your car for a red light, do these isometrics, and if you drive any distance to and from work each day, this trip alone can take care of the necessary abdominal exercises. Of course, you can also do them at your desk at the office or while you're watching TV or wherever. However, it's not wise to try them after a meal because some people find they become a little nauseated.

Chapter 20

HOW YOU CAN PREVENT
LOW BACK PROBLEMS:
The Secrets!

FOLK SAYINGS may seem trite and sound hackneyed, but you must realize they are the accumulated wisdom of thousands of years, refined and concentrated statements of what mankind has learned is the essence of truth. An ounce of prevention *is* worth a pound of cure, and where your low back is concerned, the same methods you use for prevention must also be used as part of the cure. Here then are the things you should learn, to prevent and—in part—cure any low back problems. These patterns should become part of your everyday life—at home, and at work, during all the activities of daily living from picking up a pencil to driving to your in-laws', in lifting a heavy load and for working at your desk, even in choosing your sports and your posture.

The Activities of Daily Living

If you are one of the victims of low back dysfunctions, you will just have to accept the fact that you must rethink your life if you want to avoid increasing problems and look forward to a backache-free life. The exercises outlined in the last chapter are one step on this road to a pain-free back, and you will have to find time for exercises every day—first for the corrective ones and then for some individually prescribed activity or sport.

The fundamental principle involved is to approach every activity of your daily life with essentially one thought in mind: to achieve the goal of reducing your lumbar lordosis. This necessitates changing nearly all your habitual patterns of daily living—the way you stand, walk, sit, even the way you sleep. Unfortunately, such massive change is not easy and must be gone at deliberately and systematically.

To accomplish the end of a pain-free back, you have to enter on a retraining program with a broad combination of corrective exercises and altered postural attitudes. Such a program has many pitfalls and requires constant vigilance. Even when you are willing to devote the necessary time and effort to the corrective exercises, the manner in which these are performed should be checked at intervals with your physician because patients do imperceptibly modify or embellish their performance and sometimes turn this into a harmful action instead of a helpful one.

Even when you faithfully carry out the corrective low back exercises, you may get no improvement in your low back dysfunction if there is an increased lumbar lordosis the rest of your day with all its activities. In short, you must review every single activity of your ordinary day's life to correct or alter each one so that the lordosis—the swayback—is flattened out and corrected.

Maintaining Good Low Back Posture

What is good low back posture? Essentially, if you will pull in your stomach muscles and tuck in your pelvis, you will straighten out your swayback. You can practice a proper erect posture every so often during the day—even at work. All you need do is stand unobtrusively against a wall and press your belt line against the wall, but not your head or shoulders, so that your lumbar spine forms as close to a straight up-and-down line as is comfortably possible.

To train yourself in this particular maneuver, you plant your feet twelve inches from the wall, thus making it easier for you to flatten your lumbar spine against the wall (in essence starting as with the pelvic uptilt outlined in the last chapter, where you begin with your knees flexed and work up to doing it with legs out straight). With practice you will find the lumbar-flattening maneuver can be accomplished against a wall with less and less effort, and as you get more efficient, you can gradually position your feet closer to the wall until they are against it and the exercise will do the most for your low back.

The ideal posture includes an uplifted chest so that it, not the abdomen, is the most forward part of your body. It's wise occasionally to check your posture in front of a full-length mirror; view yourself from the side just as a reminder to avoid that protruding abdomen and to substitute the uplifted chest for it. As some put it, imagine a string attached to your chest and being pulled straight up by some magic power in the ceiling.

Standing and the Bar Rail

Clearly the tavernkeepers of the last century were concerned with their livelihood and sought to protect it by installing that little brass rail; intuitively they must have known that this would permit their patrons to stand comfortably by the bar for many hours at a time. You too can learn from this little maneuver, for any time you're faced with prolonged standing you can achieve a comfortable flattening of the lumbar spine simply by placing one foot on a low stool six to eight inches high. You need only alternate the foot that's raised, from time to time, to make long standing safe for your low back.

Whenever possible, avoid prolonged standing. When this is unavoidable, use a small footstool or some object to keep one foot slightly elevated even in such daily activities as shaving or ironing, preparing food or just brushing your teeth. It's also important to move about often, not to stand in the same position for more than a few minutes. Shift from foot to foot if you should be forced to remain standing without a footstool or the like.

It's important when you stand for any length of time to avoid the very common pattern people have of leaning backwards and resting on their hands because this only exaggerates the very swayback we're trying to eliminate. To prevent this, it's even wise when standing to keep your hands in front of your body and to lean somewhat forward. And always try to remember to think often of your posture—is your pelvis tucked up under you, is your abdomen in and your chest uplifted? One trick is to imagine that you must hold a coin between your buttocks by squeezing them together; this will automatically result in a pelvic uptilt and a reduction of any lumbar lordosis.

Walking Safely

When you turn to walk from a standing posture, move your feet before you move your body so that you're not twisting; do it as a soldier would in a left or right face on the parade ground. Always avoid any jerky or sudden twisting movements. Get in the habit of opening doors widely so that you can walk comfortably without having to squeeze through. In fact, always be sure to avoid any space or situation in which you may have to assume a cramped, twisted or awkward position. Learn to move smoothly and deliberately, and be careful to avoid any jarring of your back; judge the height of curbs and steps and negotiate them deliberately and carefully.

Shoes—and Bending

The problem of high heels is now both a male and a female one, for men are making the same mistake of sacrificing health for fashion. High heels automatically result in a compensatory increase in lumbar lordosis and so should be avoided. When women feel they must wear high heels, they should avoid them during periods of prolonged standing or walking and should at least change to low heels frequently during the day and whenever possible. Men should just avoid high heels—period!

It's also best to avoid prolonged forward bending. If you have to do something for which you must get down low, use a stool to sit on, squat, or even sit on the floor, but find some way of avoiding forward bending for any length of time.

Sitting

The load thrown on the spinal disks is greater in sitting than in standing or walking, so you should learn new ways of sitting if you have a bad back. For one thing you will have to give up some of that soft living—no more of those over-stuffed chairs or sofas you can sink into so luxuriously either to read or to watch TV or just to socialize. Now it's the straight chairs with hard, firm backs and seats for you. If the chair is right, your low back will be straight and your knees should be on a level with or higher than hip joints. An excessively high chair will make your feet dangle with knees lower than hip joints, resulting in that swaybacked effect—that lumbar lordosis—we are trying so hard to avoid. If necessary, use a footstool to get your knees up and your low back straight, or, if this isn't possible, you can correct to some extent by simply crossing your knees, which also flattens out the lumbar lordosis.

It's wise not to sit too long in the same position. Get up, move about, and stretch periodically. Finally, avoid sitting on high stools.

Sleeping Protectively

Here, too, the soft life is out. A firm flat mattress with no lumps or bumps or hollows or slants is best; ideally you should have a bed board (three-quarters of an inch thick) between the mattress and spring or an orthopedic mattress. If you want to rest during the day and like to lie on your back, a pillow under your knees is best because it immobilizes and flattens your spine. At night, if you habitually sleep on your back, it's best to put a sizable blanket roll under the mattress at the level of your knees because a pillow there gets pushed away during sleep.

Sleeping on your back with your feet out straight or on your stomach is bad. The best way to sleep is to lie on your side with a low pillow under your head and your knees pulled up. You may find it most comfortable as well. Avoid lying with your arm extended above your head. If you are a victim of long-standing low back dysfunction, you may need a hospital bed with its varied adjustments for proper sleeping position.

Did Your Doctor Say "Bed Rest"?

If your doctor advises bed rest, remember this means absolute bed rest—and you can't get up every now and then, can't prop yourself up with big pillows to watch TV. Raising your body or twisting or turning puts a severe strain on an already-unhappy low back condition. *Obey your doctor*—even if he prohibits you from going to the bathroom and you have to eat your meals in bed lying on your side with a pillow under your shoulder. If you're allowed to lie on your side at other times, you may still be able to watch some TV, but otherwise it's just the radio for you.

Driving

In driving always pull your seat forward so that your knees are slightly higher than the hip joints, to keep your low back flat. Never push the seat back to the point where you're reaching for the pedals and the knees are so low that you have to sit with a swayback. Avoid driving long distances without stopping. Get out of the car and stretch at least once every hour. And *always wear* your seat belt and shoulder harness.

Lifting: It Can Be Murder on Your Back!

Lifting is one of the big culprits in finishing the job on an already-weakened low back—even lifting a pen or a paper clip. But there are rules you can follow which will protect you with any kind of heavy lifting so that you can lead a normal life:

1. Let your legs, not your back, do the work. This holds true whether it's a heavy package or a slip of paper. Bend your knees when you lift something, and never lean forward from the waist with your knees stiff. Squat in front of a heavy object, move it close to your body, and then slowly rise so that your legs and knees do the work.
2. Don't lift anything heavy without help, and then plan what each of you will do so there's no sudden load or twisting.
3. When moving an object from one place to another, shift the position of your feet and avoid any sudden twisting movements of your torso when either lifting or setting the load down.
4. Keep the object as close to your body as you can, and avoid lifting from a bent-forward position. Don't reach across furniture to open a stuck window (get up close to the window); don't reach forward to pull something out of the back seat or the trunk of your car. When you want to exert force, get close to the object.
5. Get a firm footing before lifting; a slipped foot can mean a slipped disk as well.
6. Get a firm grip on the load, preferably with your fingers completely under the object, and be sure both load and fingers are dry—moisture leads to something slipping and then a sudden twisting movement.

The Overweight Load

Being overweight usually goes along with a flabby, sagging abdomen which creates the same weight and low back problems as pregnancy. It weakens the abdominal muscles and is almost like carrying a five- or ten-pound weight around your middle whenever you're not sleeping, say, sixteen or eighteen hours a day. A normal weight and a trim figure are good protection for your low back.

The Household Hazards for Man and Woman

Every household chore—from using the vacuum cleaner to getting in and out of the car, from shoveling the snow to picking up the baby—should be looked on as a potential source of low back trouble. Do these tasks only in the light of all the instructions and approaches we've discussed and detailed. And if your back is acting up, don't try making beds or putting up the screens, doing spring cleaning or even mopping the floors. Wait until you've got the problem quiet again. The housewife might even ask her doctor about the value of wearing a girdle while doing these chores.

It's wise also to remembers the pros—the athletes who always limber up before entering a strenuous contest. You might do the same before heavy gardening or snow shoveling. Doing some of our exercises to relax and then those for the low back would likely (*if* your doctor says it's all right for *you* to do them) loosen up your muscles and lower any tension so that you won't run into trouble by overusing tight, nonelastic muscles.

You might start perhaps by just swinging a tool you're going to use—a rake or shovel, say—lazily around your head and then with increasing force. It might be wise to keep something—a sweater or jacket—handy to throw on when you've worked up a sweat so that you don't chill your back at the end of gardening. Age, too, is a factor here; as you get older, you must remember as with sports that the back tissues are less elastic and more liable to injury, so more preparation is necessary and the amount you can safely do is more limited.

The Sports Picture

Here, too, you must take a defensive profile. Bicycling, walking and swimming are wonderful conditioning exercises for your back at any age, but see that you move into them gradually; don't go out and overdo anything the first time. Sports such as golf or bowling or tennis should be approached gingerly because they involve twisting, bending and leaning, and all these actions are potentially dangerous to the low back and its disks. There is an additional risk factor in sports as we discussed in the chapter on the low back and age; as you get older, there are fewer sports you should start for the first time and more warm-up preparation is needed each time.

Back Care at Work

There are certain things to avoid at work which aren't likely to be present at home. For example, swivel chairs or chairs on rollers are to be avoided wherever possible, and so are the poorly constructed typists' chairs with a narrow back rest which tends to produce swayback.

It's also wise to work to try to change positions every half hour or so. The desk worker might type for a half hour, then do some filing or working in a different area so that the sitting alternates with walking about. It might even be possible to stand beside a table rather than sit at a desk for a while, and a low footstool or box will prevent any lumbar lordosis.

Defensive Low Back Living: Know Your Own Limits

This is vital. Recognize your age, the condition of your muscles, the amount of activity (the office worker who goes out one day a month or one vacation week a year and does violent contact sports is clearly at risk)—and the strength and condition of your low back. Learn to live within the *limits your own physical condition and age set for you;* strive for a life-style compatible with the physical realities of your body and your health.

Take all that you've learned in this book, and you can look forward to a healthy low back life, one free of pain unless you're one of those unfortunates whose musculature and disks are inherently weak. There are worse fates than not indulging in the sports or other activities that life has to offer.

So while there is a reality we can't overlook, in general and with few exceptions you may look forward to a full and comfortable life with a back that is really designed to last a lifetime—provided you give it loving, intelligent care.

SELECTED READINGS AND BIBLIOGRAPHY

"Acupuncture in America," *Medical World News* (July 19, 1974).

BARR, J. S., ET AL. "Evaluation of End Results in Treatment of Ruptured Lumbar Intervertebral Disks with Protrusion of Nucleus Pulposus," *Surgery, Gynecology and Obstetrics* (August, 1967).

BEALS, R. K., and HICKMAN, N. W. "Industrial Injuries of the Back and Extremities," *Journal of Bone and Joint Surgery* (December, 1972).

BIRK, L., ed. *Biofeedback: Behavioral Medicine.* New York: Grune & Stratton, 1973.

BLANCHARD, E. B., and YOUNG, L. D. "Clinical Applications of Biofeedback Training," *Archives of General Psychiatry* (May, 1974).

BONICA, J. J. "Therapeutic Acupuncture in the People's Republic of China," *Journal of the American Medical Association* (June 17, 1974).

———. "Acupuncture Anesthesia in the People's Republic of China," *Journal of the American Medical Association* (September 2, 1974).

"Biofeedback in Action," *Medical World News,* (March 9, 1973).

BRODIE, D. C. *Drug Utilization.* Rockville, Md.: Department of Health, Education and Welfare, 1970.

BROSS, I. D. J., and NATARAJAN, N. "Leukemia from Low Level Radiation," *New England Journal of Medicine* (July 20, 1972).

BROWN, R. F., ET AL. "Appraising Medical X-ray Protection Activities," *Practical Radiology* (April, 1973).

BUNKER, J. P. *The Anesthesiologist and the Surgeon.* Boston: Little, Brown and Company, 1972.

—— "Surgical Manpower," *New England Journal of Medicine* (January 15, 1970).

CASTELNUOVO-TEDESCO, P., and KROUT, B. M. "Psychosomatic Aspects of Chronic Pelvic Pain," *Psychiatry in Medicine,* Vol. 1, No. 2 (1970).

DUNKERLEY, G. E. "The Results of Surgery for Low Back and Leg Pain Due to Presumptive Prolapsed Intervertebral Disc," *Postgraduate Medical Journal* (February, 1971).

CARRON, H., ET AL. "Complication of Acupuncture," *Journal of the American Medical Association* (June 17, 1974).

ENGEL, G. L. "Guilt, Pain, and Success," *Psychosomatic Medicine,* Vol. XXIV, No. 1 (1962).

FARBMAN, A. A. "Neck Sprain," *Journal of the American Medical Association* (February 26, 1973).

FINNESON, B. E. *Diagnosis and Management of Pain Syndromes,* 2nd ed. Philadelphia: W. B. Saunders Company, 1969.

——. *Low Back Pain.* Philadelphia: J. B. Lippincott Company, 1973.

FORDYCE, W. E., ET AL. "Some Implications of Learning in Problems of Chronic Pain," *Journal of Chronic Disease* (1968).

FREESE, A. S. *Pain.* New York: G. P. Putnam's Sons, 1974.

HUNCKE, B. H., ET AL. "Chemonucleolysis, A Preliminary Report," to be published. *Chicago Medicine.*

"Hospital Infection," *Perspective* (2d Quarter, 1972).

Impairments Due to Injury: United States—1971. Rockville, Md.: U.S. Department of Health, Education and Welfare, December, 1973.

Independent Practitioners Under Medicare. Rockville, Md.: U.S. Department of Health, Education and Welfare, Report to Congress, 1968.

KAULMAN, C. "There Ought to be a Law Against X-ray Bunglers!" *Medical Economics* (October 23, 1972).

LEWIS, C. E. "Variations in the Incidence of Surgery," *New England Journal of Medicine* (October 16, 1969).

MARGULIS, A. R. "The Lessons of Radiobiology . . ." *American Journal of Roentgenology, Radium Therapy and Nuclear Medicine* (April, 1973).

McCLENAHAN, J. L. "Wasted X-rays," *Radiology* (August, 1970).

MEAD, B. T. "Women's Complaints with Sexual Connotations," *Medical Aspects of Human Sexuality* (April, 1972).

MILLER, R. G., and BURTON, R. "Stroke Following Chiropractic Manipulation of the Spine," *Journal of the American Medical Association* (July 8, 1974).

ODOM, G. L. "Neurological Surgery in Our Changing Times," *Journal of Neurosurgery* (September, 1972).

Prevalence of Chronic Skin and Musculoskeletal Conditions. United States—1969. Rockville, Md.: U.S. Department of Health, Education and Welfare, August 1974.

"Reassessment of Surgical Specialties in the United States," *Archives of Surgery* (June, 1972).

Report of the Committee on Chymopapain. Chicago, Ill.: American Academy of Orthopaedic Surgeons.

Report of the National Advisory Commission on Health Manpower, Vol. II. Rockville, Md.: U.S. Department of Health, Education and Welfare, November, 1967.

RIGGS, B. L. Report on combination therapy for Osteoporosis, given on November 3, 1973, before American Rheumatism Association (Arthritis Foundation).

RUSKIN, A. Report on relationship between back trauma and impotence given at American Congress of Rehabilitation Medicine, January, 1972.

RYAN, E. D., and KOVACIC, C. R. "Pain Tolerance and Athletic Participation," *Perceptual and Motor Skills* (1966).

SHEALY, C. N. "Facets in Back and Sciatic Pain," *Minnesota Medicine* (March, 1974).

————, and MAURER, D. "Transcutaneous Nerve Stimulation for Control of Pain, *Surgical Neurology* (January, 1974).

STERNBACH, R. A., ET AL. "Traits of Pain Patients . . ." *Psychosomatics* (July–August, 1973).

STEWART, R. B., and CLUFF, L. E. "Studies on the Epidemiology of Adverse Drug Reactions . . ." *The Johns Hopkins Medical Journal* (December, 1971).

"Specialties Divide on Drug for Back Pain," *Medical World News* (September 13, 1974).

WILTSE, L. L. "Chymopapain in the Treatment of Disc Disease." Paper presented before Section on Neurological Surgery, Annual Convention of American Medical Association, June 24, 1974.

INDEX